The Essential
Homebirth Guide

The Essential Homebirth Guide

For Families Planning or Considering Birthing at Home

Jane E. Drichta, CPM
and Jodilyn Owen, CPM

With Foreword by Dr. Christiane Northrup

Gallery Books

New York   London   Toronto   Sydney   New Delhi

G

Gallery Books
A Division of Simon & Schuster, Inc.
1230 Avenue of the Americas
New York, NY 10020

First Gallery Books trade paperback edition February 2013

GALLERY BOOKS and colophon are registered trademarks of Simon & Schuster, Inc.

For information about special discounts for bulk purchases, please contact Simon & Schuster Special Sales at 1-866-506-1949 or business@simonandschuster.com.

The Simon & Schuster Speakers Bureau can bring authors to your live event. For more information or to book an event contact the Simon & Schuster Speakers Bureau at 1-866-248-3049 or visit our website at www.simonspeakers.com.

Designed by Davina Mock-Maniscalco

Manufactured in the United States of America

10 9 8 7 6 5 4 3 2 1

Library of Congress Cataloging-in-Publication Data
Drichta, Jane E.
    The essential homebirth guide : for families planning or considering birthing at home / Jane E. Drichta and Jodilyn Owen ; with foreword by Dr. Christiane Northrup.
        p. cm.
    1. Childbirth at home—Handbooks, manuals, etc.
I. Owen, Jodilyn. II. Title.
    RG661.5.E88 2013
    618.2—dc23   2012034691

ISBN 978-1-4516-6862-9
ISBN 978-1-4516-6863-6 (ebook)

Contents

"The only ones who truly know your story are the ones who helped you write it."

—unknown

Dedicated with love to our families, who started us on this journey, sustained us as we walked, and rejoiced with us through it all.

Foreword

by Christiane Northrup, MD,
author of *Women's Bodies, Women's Wisdom*

GIVING BIRTH TRANSFORMS A woman at a cellular level. Laboring and birthing with your inner guidance and power fully intact has the potential to open wellsprings of wisdom within you that you hadn't known existed. When I first witnessed a birth as a medical student, this power filled the room. And I nearly fell to my knees weeping at the beauty of it. And so, as a board-certified ob-gyn who has been at the forefront of holistic health for women for decades, and at the bedside of countless birthing women, I wanted to stand up and cheer for this book!

I was an ob-gyn resident when electronic fetal monitoring was introduced. And though fetal monitoring has never been scientifically shown to do anything except lead to more interventions, this unquestioned technology is now standard in all hospital births. The c-section rate after its introduction soared to 25 percent almost overnight. Though most of us thought *that* was too high at the time, the new U.S. rate of 30 to 50 percent of all births via c-section is simply unacceptable. Unfortunately, this same rate is now common in many countries besides the United States. I have been dismayed to see how quickly women have been willing to turn their power over to the system. But I also know how deeply ingrained the fear of childbirth is. And how adversely affected most women are by the media depiction of what is meant to be a natural and empowering process. It is no wonder that the maternal mortality rate has doubled in the United States in the last twenty years. No matter how good your intentions, you simply can't fool with a natural process (birth) that much and expect Mother Nature to sit quietly by and not warn you!

But over the past few years, this inexorable tide of intervention has begun to change. Today's women are claiming their birthing power in droves. (Many, like me, attempted this in the 1970s and '80s, but the cultural support for doing so was not nearly as robust as it is now.) Today's women, often with baby boomer mothers who were pioneers in the natural birth movement themselves, are bringing their bodies into alignment with their minds and their emotions. They are remembering that they have the innate ability to birth safely and joyfully. They are waking up to the fact that hospitals and the mind-sets that run them too often interfere with normal birth—despite the best intentions of the staff.

Individuals such as Ricki Lake, and her incredible film *The Business of Being Born*, and of course the legendary midwife Ina May Gaskin, whose safety record in birth is unparalleled, are part of this exciting movement toward full-scale female empowerment—which includes the wisdom of the body.

Deep in my soul, I have always been a midwife disguised as an MD. I know what it's like to truly attend a birth—standing by while a woman goes deeply into herself to see what she is really capable of. And I have had two children of my own—both naturally without drugs or epidurals, though in a hospital. If I had it to do over again, I would birth at home. I would have done so then, except for the fact that there was so little support that I don't know how I would have pulled it off and kept my standing in my profession. Today we have statistics that have proved, beyond any shadow of a doubt, that homebirth for low-risk women is as safe as birth in the hospital. And in many cases, even safer!

Into this fertile soil of new birth beginnings, Jane Drichta and Jodilyn Owen have brought what I consider the absolute *bible* of birth preparation. *The Essential Homebirth Guide* is for *every* pregnant woman—whether or not she plans to have a homebirth. This book lays out the ways in which the midwifery model is true partnership care—as opposed to the medical "we will save you" model, the one with the unfortunate side effect of a woman abdicating her power to an outer authority, thus forgetting her own. This guide reads like a trusted and skilled friend. Just check out the table of contents. It covers everything you need to know—from low iron to what to do if you are diagnosed with beta strep.

Most delightfully of all, this incredible manual gives you the tools that you need to access your inner birthing wisdom—and to truly trust yourself. The essence of self-esteem and personal power is self-trust. And the trust in your body that birthing provides will guide you for the rest of your life. And also, of course, provide an atmosphere of love and bonding for your new baby. The authors say it best: "When mothers look back at their pregnancies and birth and feel that they were pivotal players at decision points, they feel filled with a positive and energetic power. That power is not in the method, geography, provider, or location of your care or birth. It is within you and comes forward as you take an active leading role in your care and birth. Midwifery care recognizes this, and our explanation of this kind of care gives you another great tool to take with you as you move forward."

Amen, sisters.

Welcome

WELCOME! WE ARE SO pleased that you are investigating home-birth and that you have found this resource. More families than ever are making the intentional, educated decision to receive midwifery care and birth at home. As birth practitioners and educators, we have sat with hundreds of women as they searched their hearts to make informed decisions about their pregnancies and births. We know it can be an overwhelming experience to sift through and decipher all of the information available in a meaningful way.

While each pregnancy and birth is unique, we tend to hear the same questions over and over again. We have answered these questions in a variety of ways over the years—through lists of good Web sites or books, prewritten e-mails, pamphlets, and handouts. We've created and participated in online groups for homebirth families to ask and answer each other's questions. We've considered walking around Seattle with sandwich boards and megaphones, or hiring a plane to skywrite some of the answers. These methods evolved over the years but our goal was always to get quality information into parents' hands.

It has been our privilege to work with mothers and fathers who are seeking knowledge, partners in care, and healthy, meaningful pregnancy and birth experiences. We are thrilled to offer you this resource, so that you can now open one book and find plenty of information delivered through the lens of trust in birth, mothers, babies, and families.

We know that as expecting parents, you are trying to find your way through a sea of information, research, and opinion. This book is full of all three. Our goal is not to persuade you to choose the midwifery model of care or a homebirth. Our goal is not to rescue you or save you or have you crying out after your birth, "I couldn't have done it without you!" Our goal is to open your range of experience and exposure, so that when you make decisions regarding where and how to birth, you will be making truly informed ones. We consider ourselves guides on one path open to expectant mothers and their families. Take a look around, ask questions, and enjoy the view.

There is an abundance of material available about hospital-based prenatal care and birthing. Read it, digest it. Read this book and others about out-of-hospital birth. Talk to your partner and people you trust. There is no one hard-and-fast way to figure out the best kind of care for your pregnancy or birth. Where you start may not be where you end, and your process may lead you through several providers before you find the perfect match.

After years of working with hundreds of women, we can say emphatically that there is one character trait that we have seen lead to success in birthing: flexibility. Flexibility leads to the kind of success that is priceless and immeasurable. Some people define a good birth in simple terms: physically healthy mother and physically healthy baby. We certainly believe in healthy mothers and babies, but it also runs much deeper than that. As you cradle your newborn in your arms, you should know deep in your soul that all of the thousands of decisions you made to get to this moment were yours. Knowing the depth of that truth, you can work backward. What kind of care, what kind of support team, and what kind of information do you need so that you can reach that moment?

When mothers look back at their pregnancies and birth and feel that they were pivotal players at decision points, they feel filled with a positive and energetic power. That power is not in the method, geography, provider, or location of your care or birth. It is within you and comes forward as you take an active leading role in your care and birth. Midwifery care recognizes this, and our explanation of this kind of care gives you another great tool to take with you as you move forward.

You are on a journey to birth your baby: a child of your family, a member of society, a whole human being who will contribute to our world. We hope this journey is steeped in knowledge and self-awareness as you come into your mother-self. This book is all about how capable, healthy, and strong mothers and babies can be when they work together.

We have called upon the wisdom of the midwives who came before us, our teachers and mentors, our colleagues, the families we have worked with, and the researchers and scientists of our time to address the issues that current-day families are facing when it comes to prenatal care and birth. Through sharing these experiences and insights, we hope to see more mothers in the moments after birth gazing into their newborn's eyes and crying out, *"We did it!"*

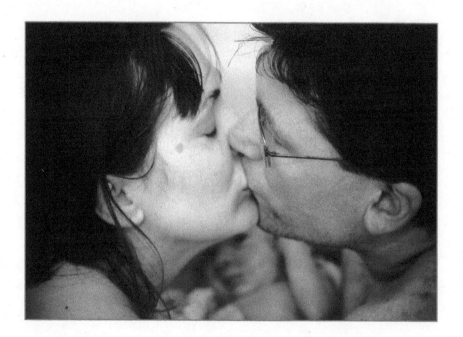

A Note from the Authors

WORKING TOGETHER IS WHAT this book is all about. Babies do best when they are birthed into strong, intentional families, and these families can take many forms. We have had the privilege to work with so many families and individuals over the years: married, partnered, single parents, adopting parents, straight, gay, or polyamorous. While we try to use language that reflects this, oftentimes we revert to the traditional mother/father dyad. Please know that this is purely for semantic reasons, and does not reflect how we practice. Similarly, we know several wonderful male midwives and doulas. But rather than use the cumbersome "she/he" construction, we have defaulted to female.

What you won't find in this book are chapters and chapters of high-risk care solutions. We have written this book to meet the needs of homebirthing women, and these women are by definition low risk. We do detail common conditions that you may encounter, but none of them will automatically rule you out of a homebirth. There are plenty of resources out there for families who face serious medical challenges, and we encourage you to take advantage of them if the need arises. If you risk out of homebirth and require extensive testing, treatment, or bed rest, we encourage you to check out Appendix D: Resources for Higher Risk Mamas with Homebirth Hearts.

We also do not go into great detail about each individual test you may be offered. Each midwife has her own set of laboratory work that she routinely orders, and will go over the tests with you as the need arises. New ones are developed all the time. Technology marches on!

And finally, we are so grateful to the dozens of women and families who have shared their stories with us. We have almost exclusively changed the names to protect the privacy of the families and providers who worked with them and in some cases where we had several similar stories, we consolidated them to illustrate a certain topic or idea.

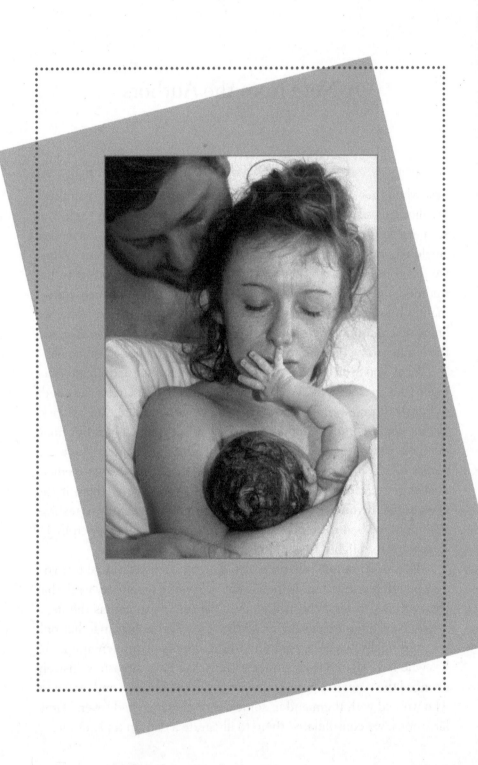

CHAPTER ONE

The Story of Homebirth

- The history of homebirth
- Modern homebirth
- The anatomy of homebirth today

MAMA SAYS

The day before Evelyn's birth, I walked several miles around our small town by the ocean. The leaves were fallen and crisp on the sidewalk. The wind was strong, and pressed my jacket onto my heavy belly. I remember literally gasping at the beauty of that day, that walk, that moment in time: the red leaves of a Japanese maple against the blue autumn sky, the woolly backs of sheep in a field, the smell of wood smoke in the air. There is something about the end of pregnancy that opens a woman to the earth, the universe. Perhaps it is standing at the edge, waiting, waiting for one to become two.

—Ashley

The History of Homebirth

ALL THE BEST STORIES start with "Once upon a time," and this one is no exception. Scarcely longer than a breath, this phrase takes us outside our regular, everyday existence and places us squarely in the middle of Somewhere Else. This Somewhere can be real or imaginary, familiar or foreign; it doesn't matter in the least. For stories deal in truth, and our hearts recognize and respond readily to truth. It is a consequence of being human, and one of our greatest strengths. Well, that and birthing our babies.

Like babies, stories come by us, and through us. Both are supreme acts of creation and creativity. This story, "The Tale of Western Homebirth Midwifery," is filled with contention and controversy, politics and death. It's a thriller, to be sure, and it doesn't even have an ending yet. Some of its major characters probably haven't even been born. It is a grand story, epic in scope, and every family who makes the choice to birth at home has a role in it.

Once upon a time, there was a midwife named Bridget Lee Fuller. She has the distinction of being the first European midwife in the New World. She sailed on the *Mayflower*, where she assisted with the births of two pregnant women on board. Mrs. Fuller later settled in Plymouth, Massachusetts, where, in exchange for her work, she received a house and a generous stipend from the town. This is hardly the stereotypical persecuted witch midwife of lore. In fact, there is ample evidence that at the beginning of the colonial period, midwives were respected members of society and were highly esteemed.

These women were usually not formally trained, although the earliest English colonists most likely included some educated women. (There were midwifery licensing procedures in England as early as the seventeenth century, authorized by the Church, forbidding witchcraft, and encouraging the midwife to tend the poor.) These early midwives relied heavily on folk remedies, herbal preparations, and experience. Women could expect ergot for labor pain, or belladonna to prevent a threatened miscarriage. And they seemed to have remarkably good outcomes. Contrary to popular belief, the leading cause of death for colonial women was not childbirth, but disease.[1]

Martha Ballard, a midwife working in rural Maine between 1785 and 1812, left a detailed diary of her midwifery exploits and daily life. For twenty-seven years, she faithfully recorded visits to and from her neighbors, the weather, and the other minutiae that make up an ordinary life. (For more information on Martha Ballard, please read *A Midwife's Tale* by Laurel Thatcher Ulrich.) Over the course of her career, she recorded one maternal death for every 198 live births, about .5 percent.[2] Around 1930, when about half of the births in America took place in the hospital, the maternal death rate was about .7 percent and the infant death rate was 1.9 percent. Ballard's infant mortality rate was similarly low, about 1.8 percent.

So how did the community midwife go from being a valued professional to being seen as a dangerously uneducated witch, suitable for attending only the most disenfranchised members of society?

Midwifery is one of a handful of professions that combines hand work, head work, and heart work. As such, it can be difficult to understand from the outside. Being able to stop a woman from bleeding to death or help a baby start breathing are easily measurable skills. If the midwife does them correctly, the baby and mother live. If she does not, they die or suffer lasting repercussions.

It was the other two legs of the proverbial birthing stool, the work of the head and the heart that sometimes led to trouble. Women were largely denied formal education in these early days, and sometimes seemed (to their male counterparts) to have too much knowledge—if such a thing is possible. They did their work mostly at night, with very few people around, using gifts from the earth herself: the herbs and native plants of the surrounding countryside. Their work was warm and moist, dark and internal, quiet and secret. This powerful feminine archetype was very threatening in a patriarchal society, which generally accepted that power, morality, and wisdom flowed from God to kings to noblemen and then spread to the rest of society. How could these midwives, these women, be privy to the literal secrets of life and death? What was going on? If this knowledge didn't come from

God—and it obviously had not, as it had clearly bypassed the kings and noblemen—then it must have come from the devil.

Along with this apparent supernatural collaboration, midwives were also beginning to have other problems by the early nineteenth century, this time technological and economic in nature. Two hundred years earlier, the Chamberlain family "invented" the obstetrical forceps.[3] (Perhaps it is better to say that they improved on an ancient design, and began to use them frequently. Crude versions had been used by eleventh-century Arabian doctors.[4]) The Chamberlains kept their design secret from other doctors of the time, presumably so that they could have a monopoly in the market, but eventually word leaked out. More and more doctors began using these instruments, improving on their design, and publicizing their results.

As the use of forceps increased, maternal mortality rates improved drastically enough that William Leishman, writing in 1873, referred to the forceps as, "The Great Prime Mover of Obstetrics. . . . It is scarcely possible to exaggerate the importance of this instrument, which is simple in construction, easy of application, and marvelous in power."[5] As the years went by, infant mortality rates began to fall as doctors became more skilled in their use.

So where were the midwives during this period? Well, they certainly were not in lecture halls or medical school. They were doing what they had always done, catching babies. However, they were doing it without the benefit of this new technology, and they were doing it in people's homes, not in the newly opened obstetrical wards. It was becoming a status symbol to deliver with a doctor, with his instruments and, by 1847, chloroform for anesthesia. On April 7 of that year, Henry Wadsworth Longfellow's wife, Fanny, became the first woman to inhale the gas during childbirth.[6] Her labor lasted five and a half hours, and she was apparently very satisfied with the experiment. Between her experience and that of Queen Victoria birthing with the drug in 1853, childbirth, at least for the famous and well-to-do, was rapidly becoming a spectator sport, something others did to you, rather than something needing any direct participation from the mother. By the advent of the Industrial Revolution, in both England

and America, the upper classes saw the traditional midwife as dirty, uneducated, and thoroughly unmodern.

This attitude persisted through most of the twentieth century. Technology continued to advance, with vacuum extractors and epidurals, and the once-always-fatal cesarean section worked its way toward being the most common surgical procedure performed in the United States. Early feminists applauded the routine use of spinal anesthesia, claiming it was their right to birth without pain. And the American homebirth midwife faded further and further into the background.

Our country's history of midwifery largely rests with the "granny midwives" who practiced in America from the early 1700s through the late 1800s. They were predominantly African-American women, and functioned as birth attendants and healers. The stewardship of this important community role was often passed down matrilineally, with long apprenticeships that only ended when the senior midwife retired or passed away. As the medical establishment grew in their practice of obstetrics and nurse-midwifery, granny midwives became the target of social and professional persecution. Just as the obstetricians feared the white midwives' knowledge and abilities, so too with the granny midwives. Physicians lobbied for restrictive legislation against granny midwives and drove this culture underground and eventually to extinction. Prior to this time African-American women, like women in so many cultures around the world, held positions of respect as healers and particularly midwives within their communities. The book *Folks Do Get Born* by Marie Campbell was compiled and organized by a group of granny midwives in rural Georgia and published in 1946. It is a firsthand account of the life and history of granny midwives in America.

Modern Homebirth

DURING THE LATE 1960S and early 1970s, things began to shift. Against the backdrop of free love, Vietnam, Kent State, and flower children, childbearing women gradually began to gather their own power. Change was slow in coming, as change often is. After all, life was so busy! The burgeoning Equal Rights movement, the withdrawal of our troops from Southeast Asia, not to mention just going to work and paying bills . . . it took time for mothers to realize that something so mundane, so normal, as having a baby could be so important.

And this is where some women realized that they had a problem. Women had been so disconnected from birth for so many years that the medicalized version *was* normal. In the 1950s, women went to the hospital, were put to sleep using scopolamine, and hours later, woke up a mother. In the 1970s, women went to the hospital and were given a spinal anesthetic or pudendal block (a technique used to numb the vaginal and rectal areas). Women went to the hospital. It was just what they did. Until it wasn't.

No discussion of recent homebirthing would be complete without mentioning Ina May Gaskin. This unassuming English major left her home in California with a group of likeminded folks and caravanned across America in search of a place to build a community. They dreamed of a place where people could live close to the land, feeding themselves from the soil, worshipping as they saw fit, and birthing their babies into an atmosphere of love, respect, and joy. The group found their new home outside of Summertown, Tennessee, and in 1971 The Farm was born. Ina May received some rudimentary midwifery training during their journey, during which several pregnant women gave birth, so as the group settled into their new lives, she enlisted a local doctor to teach her more skills. This was the beginning.

In 1976 Ina May's first book, *Spiritual Midwifery*, was published. Part childbirth manual, part birth-story anthology, this book was the first to unapologetically state that babies could be born safely and happily at home. It presented homebirth in an accessible way, using plain language and lots and lots of stories. It spoke to women in their own language, and women listened.

Spiritual Midwifery validated what many women were beginning to suspect: that perhaps they would be better off to feel the sensations and acknowledge that while birth hurt, it was also very powerful. This time in the history of birth was part of the tipping point when women expressed and claimed their power in society. Birth was intimately connected to self-perception, and entire new paradigms across westernized cultures bloomed out of this awareness. With power, women could determine their futures both personally and professionally. While seizing upon these ideas and experiences may have felt dangerous, some women were not afraid. They flipped their feathered hair defiantly, marched themselves right into their homes, and birthed their babies.

The Anatomy of Homebirth Today

MOTHERS AND MIDWIVES WHO partake in homebirth today have arrived here through the work of thousands of years of other mothers and midwives. Approximately 1 percent of all American babies are born outside of the hospital, and that number is growing every year.[7] Homebirth is an old idea, but women have reclaimed and reinvented it. Midwives are back. They are educated, well trained, and full of energy for birth and all of the power it brings into the lives of the families they work with. So this brings us to the present day, with modern parents and modern midwives. Just who is birthing at home in America today? According to a study done in 1995, homebirthing mothers tend to have less formal education, identify as Caucasian, and are pregnant with their second or subsequent child. They are not likely to drink or smoke during pregnancy. They begin prenatal care later, and are less likely to do all routine testing. Additionally, their baby's health is likely to be better than the average American baby's.[8]

Today mothers over thirty still make up the majority of homebirthers, and they are extremely well versed in the language and technicalities of childbirth. Many of these women are professionals, with years of formal education behind them. They approach childbirth as they would any other project. It is not uncommon for these women to walk into their midwifery appointments carrying the latest studies, eager to discuss and debate them. Homebirth midwives love this! It's a great opportunity to get to know what aspects of childbirth you are drawn to and to really personalize your care.

Even if they do not have advanced degrees or high-powered jobs, homebirth moms still tend to know an awful lot about having babies. These women know the birthing options in their community intimately, and have identified what setting and provider best matches their personal birthing philosophy. They also are aware of all their birthing resources, and feel like they can exercise any option that they might need.

> By the time I decided to have children, I had attended many hospital births as a doula, and worked with families as a childbirth and lactation educator. I knew there had to be a better way. While I witnessed several beautiful, empowering births in that setting, I saw many more that started with educated, strong parents giving their birth experience over to the medical staff. I wanted my birth experience to be respected as the unique event that it was.
>
> Also, I didn't want to be treated like I was embarking on a journey fraught with risk and peril, even though I was a geezer at thirty-six years old.
>
> My husband and I decided that a homebirth was the right choice for us. We live in a city with some great hospitals, and we figured if events required medical intervention, we were a short car ride, or even a walk, away. We ended up exercising that option with our first baby, who was born at the hospital after a long exhausting labor, but we had an amazing birth at home with our second.
>
> —Elisabeth

Elisabeth's story brings to light one of the most common reasons for homebirthing: the feeling that birth is not a medical event, and should not be treated as one.

In other areas of their lives, many homebirth families utilize alternative therapies such as naturopathic medicine, massage therapy, and acupuncture, while some families use strictly allopathic care for their medical needs. However, both see birth as natural, and potentially life changing, and seek out a location that can support this vision.

Anecdotally speaking, around 2003 I started to see high-powered (business-owner or upper-management), professional, thirty-five-plus-year-old clients seek homebirth in droves. Sometimes I would meet them, and watching them with their planners and heels (no flats for these fashion-forward mamas!), I thought I had landed in the twilight zone. But after really talking with them, and after I had so many clients like this, I learned something. These women considered themselves great decision makers and team leaders. They had run corporations, managed huge divisions, or litigated very public cases successfully. The homebirth model spoke to them. They built their team and gathered their resources, collecting wisdom and knowledge from us. Smart and savvy, this new crop of homebirth mothers brought homebirth out of the hippie/indie crowd and into mainstream, Main Street U.S.A.

—Claire (certified labor doula)

For some, homebirth is an economic decision. For the underinsured, and those with no coverage at all, homebirth makes financial sense. It is far cheaper to birth with an out-of-hospital provider than in a hospital with its lab fees, provider payments, facility charges, and so forth. For those paying out of pocket, the average homebirth costs between $2,000 and $5,000, depending on location. Many times this is even less costly than a hospital birth with insurance, once you add up the co-pays and charges your insurance doesn't cover.

I am a single mom and self-employed. I have a college degree and come from a stable, loving home. I live in a suburb of a major metropolitan area and own my own home. At the time of my first pregnancy, I had not been able to afford health insurance. Homebirth made sense to me for a bunch of reasons, but I certainly would not have been able to afford prenatal care and a hospital birth out of pocket. I mean, I wanted to be able to eat too! I'm superhealthy, and live an active lifestyle, so I felt I had a really good shot at having a great homebirth. And I did!

—Beth

For people with insurance, homebirth can also make economic sense, although it does depend on where you live. Some states require insurance plans to pay for homebirth and some do not. Several states, such as Washington and New Mexico, currently also provide Medicaid coverage for homebirth. Brenda thought that she was ineligible for insurance coverage for her homebirth:

I'm a massage therapist who lives in a suburb of a major city. Our family is middle income, Caucasian, and I was definitely the first of my friends to investigate homebirth. I spent several hours on the phone with our insurance company trying to find out if homebirth was even covered. The outsourced call center employee was unable to help me. I kept at them, demanding to speak to a manager. After several phone calls I finally got them to send me a letter stating that they would indeed cover my homebirth! I found this whole problem quite bizarre as the cost of my planned homebirth was about $13,000 less than the cost of a planned hospital birth.

My first baby was born in 2001 at an out-of-hospital birth center, and I've had two more at home since then. I really wanted to avoid the use of pain medications in labor, since I react badly to them. I took an active role in my prenatal care and always felt I was given the option to gather and question information. From these experiences I learned how to ask for and interpret information. The time I spent with my midwives gave me skills and tools that I use throughout my life. I attribute many of my strengths to the work I did during my pregnancies and early mothering, thanks to the midwifery model of care and homebirth.

Some families choose homebirth out of a deep religious conviction. They believe that God made women's bodies to bear children, that the design is perfect, and that children need not be born in a technological environment. They trust that the birthing process is divinely inspired and draw great strength from this.

I believe homebirth is a safe and wonderful way to bring a child into this world. I also feel that women have robbed themselves of one of the Heavenly Father's greatest expressions of womanhood and joy by allowing the hospital to invade this most private and sacred part of a woman's life. There are times when a hospital and doctors are necessary, and I am so grateful to know they are there for the emergencies.

After I had my first baby in the hospital, I realized I could have a better experience and that God created women to have babies! Of course there are medical exceptions, but it makes more sense to work with the body's natural process than to constantly interfere with it. My homebirths were some of the most wonderful experiences I had ever had!

—Sarah

One of the fastest growing segments of the homebirthing population is those who have had a previous birth in the hospital and left feeling disrespected, battered, or hurt. This trauma can be severe and long-lasting, and has led many women to birth at home. The type of behavior described in Diana's story below is the opposite of gentle, respectful maternity care and can never be condoned, regardless of location.

We decided to do a homebirth for our second child because we had a really terrible hospital experience with our first. We arrived at the hospital and the intake nurse looked at me and said, "Who are you? Who sent you here?" in an angry, accusing way. That set the tone for all of the staff interactions we had; they were overbusy and didn't have a room for me for twenty-four hours.

I labored alone that first twenty-four hours in the triage area, with a small bed and no room to move. I had tested positive for strep B so they started an IV and gave me antibiotics every four hours. By the next day, after six bags of antibiotics, I had a raging yeast infection. When the baby finally came, his skin was colonized by the yeast, and the hospital whisked him off to the Neonatal Intensive Care Unit (NICU). They thought it was herpes. Neither my husband nor I have herpes. They put him on antivirals. The dermatologist said it was yeast, but once they started the antivirals, it was hospital policy to continue the forty-eight-hour course.

So, he started life hooked up to some pretty harsh drugs and separated from me. My milk didn't come in for weeks. Meanwhile, since the NICU unit understood that this baby wasn't actually sick, they stopped monitoring him, and his IV came loose and the meds burned his wrist and arm. He's seven now and still has the scars. On day five, they finally let us take him home. We had a lot of trouble with nursing, and separation anxiety so intense that I ended up leaving my job because he couldn't handle daycare. He continues to have separation anxiety. We can't help but wonder if it comes from this early hospital experience imprinting this powerful message.

So, that's why we had a homebirth! Our midwives were lovely, and they handled the new baby so gently and reverently for his first exam; it was such a contrast to the rough treatment we all received at the hospital. Homebirth is not for everyone, but it was best for us.

—Diana

Whatever your reason for considering homebirth, you are in good company. More women than ever before are seeking the many benefits that out-of-hospital midwifery care provides. A new paradigm for maternity care is rising up, and we are excited that you are part of this story.

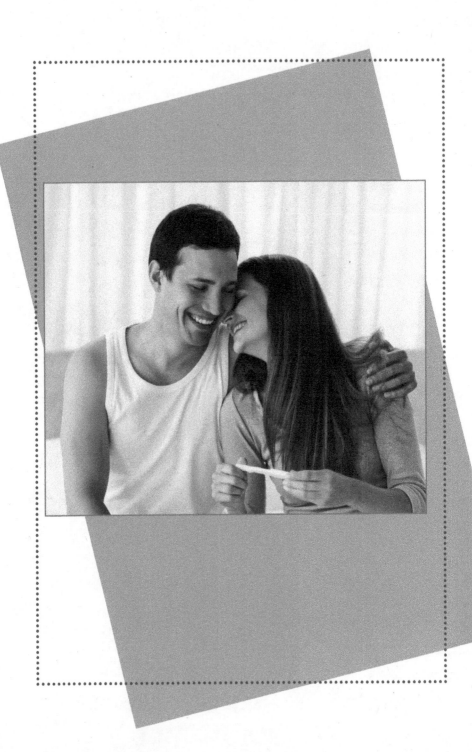

CHAPTER TWO

The Journey Begins

- You're pregnant!
- Choosing a homebirth provider and establishing care
- Prenatal nutrition

MAMA SAYS

The greatest gift I have received in my life as a result of my homebirth, after my beautiful son, is the transformative force it has created in my life. Because I was able to birth the way I wanted to and to journey through the entire birth process naturally, I now have the embodied knowledge that I can truly *do anything*!

I feel so much more willing to try new things, to attempt to do things that may have scared me before or to try things and not really care anymore about whether or not I might fail. I experience the change in myself every day!

—Taylor

You're Pregnant!

My husband and I had been trying to conceive without success for two years. I had experienced several months where I thought I was pregnant but the tests came back negative.

I was on a business trip and felt extremely tired, my breasts were sore, and I felt ravenously hungry. I tried not to get excited, but it was hard to ignore my hopes. When I got home, I told my husband how I was feeling. He did not want to see me suffer again so we agreed to wait for a few days before buying a test.

I finally went to the supermarket and bought a test. Every baby and child seemed to jump out at me, and I felt lonely, and scared that I would never be able to conceive. When we got home, I took some deep breaths and peed on the test. I watched the seconds tick away and then looked and saw the word "Pregnant." I was shocked. I was shaking and ran out to the kitchen and put the test on the counter in front of my husband. He clearly thought I was upset, and he gave me a hug and said, "It's okay, it's okay." I held the stick up so he would look at it and see that word "Pregnant."

His eyes flew open and he held me close to him. We cried together and then spent the day relaxing and in a dreamlike state. That night he had a big talk with my belly. It was a great day to share with him.

—Anne

When you find out you are carrying a baby, it can feel like the pause at the top of a roller coaster just before it plummets down a giant hill—a sort of suspended thrill where you lose track of everything, except your breath catching in your throat. Whether this space in time is followed by euphoria, disbelief, fear, or hysteria will depend on your own circumstances. One thing is certain: your life will never be the same. The experience of suddenly transitioning from individual self to self-with-other is profound. No wonder it is hard to talk straight, breathe, or swallow. This is just as true for the pregnancy that is longed for and worked for as one that is a surprise.

A woman often experiences a rapid-fire sequence of events—from discovering she is pregnant, to realizing she is the only being who can nurture this new life, to wondering what she "should be doing" in this instant to take care of her baby. Take a deep breath and relax, while we tackle your early pregnancy questions.

When is the best time to test for pregnancy?

TODAY WOMEN LEARN ABOUT their pregnancy—a very physical event—in a very intellectual way. With the advent of sensitive home pregnancy tests, women know as early as a few days before the missed period. This is a huge change from how women learned of their pregnancies even fifty years ago. Historically, missing your period was considered a reliable indicator, but some first-time mothers were not completely sure until they felt their baby move, around twenty weeks or so.

As hard as it is to wait, we are designed to come into this knowledge slowly, through an awareness of changes and sensations in our body. There is a purpose to the *process* of pregnancy and birthing, which transcends technology. It pushes us to new understanding about the meaning of time, patience, acceptance, and control. It is a time of awakening and of growth—from *woman* into *mother.*

It is usually around seven to fourteen days after a missed period that the first recognizable symptoms may be present for a woman who has conceived. Each pregnancy is best understood by the pregnant woman. It's important to pay attention to the body and all of its changes and messages. This can be easier to do if you can hold off on testing for a few days. That said, if you have been trying to conceive and are eager to know, it is hard to wait! We have had calls from many women who took a pregnancy test shortly after a missed period and were thrilled beyond belief to see the second line darken. We have also had calls from many women who have been feeling sensations of pregnancy for weeks and want to come in to confirm their suspicions. The ideal time for peeing on a stick? When you are ready to!

How late is too late to confirm my pregnancy?

WE HAVE ALL HEARD the stories and seen the television shows about those women who didn't know they were pregnant until they delivered, so clearly, it's never really too late. However, if you are interested in genetic testing, or have reason to be interested in termination, it does behoove you to see a provider as soon as possible. Also, there are certain nutritional elements that do their best work early in your pregnancy. If you are trying to conceive, it makes sense to be taking a good-quality prenatal vitamin, which includes folic acid, other B vitamins, and a reasonable amount of iron.

What symptoms should I look for if I suspect I am pregnant?

THERE ARE LOADS OF variations on the themes here, but generally speaking you can expect to feel the following:

- I didn't get my period!
  - *There may be cramping sensations but no bleeding.*
- My boobs are big!
  - *Breasts are full or feel heavy, tingly, tender, or achy.*
- I have to pee (again)!
  - *Frequent urination or the overwhelming need to pee is common.*
- I keep falling asleep.
  - *The need to sleep, often described as "fatigue," is all encompassing.*

- I have the urge to swoon, like they did in the old black-and-white movies when a woman found out she was in "the family way."

  + *Lightheadedness is very common, although very few women actually faint.*

- My husband's cologne is revolting!

  + *Most pregnant women have a heightened sense of smell.*

- Ewwww.

  + *That's a technical term for "suddenly something doesn't agree with me"—foods, odors, sights, or even thoughts that never bothered you before can make you queasy, want to puke, or set off your gag reflex faster than you ever thought possible.*

So, am I pregnant?

TODAY'S DRUG, GROCERY, AND even superstore brands of pregnancy tests are as efficient as any urine test a midwife or physician has access to. They all measure the amount of human chorionic gonadotropin, commonly known as HcG, in the urine. Besides the signs we call presumptive listed above, there are signs we call probable and positive that can confirm a pregnancy and include these:

- positive blood or urine test
- changes in the shape and size of the uterus
- the ability to feel the baby in the uterus from the outside
- fluttering in the belly, which is the sensation of movement a pregnant mother feels between eighteen and twenty-two weeks of pregnancy
- the cervix softens and takes on a blueish color (visible during a vaginal exam)

- the presence of fetal heart tones heard through a stethoscope or Doppler or seen on an ultrasound

- visual confirmation that there is a baby en utero through the use of ultrasound

---

Choosing a Homebirth Provider and Establishing Care

Pregnancy confirmed. Now what?!

FIRST, TAKE A BREATH! Give yourself a hug and say something nice in the mirror, such as, "You will be great at this!" You are your own best expert (a theme we will revisit time and time again) and you *will* be able to do this. We promise! Now, it's your job to do your research, access your intuition, and find yourself a great provider.

Deciding upon a provider is more than choosing a practitioner (or practice) to care for you during your pregnancy. This decision will determine your birthing options and will set the tone for the style of maternity care you receive.

When should I have my first prenatal visit?

TYPICALLY, THE FIRST PRENATAL visit happens between 9 and 12 weeks of pregnancy, but you can schedule this visit any time after you have missed your period. You can also start the process of interviewing a provider before you conceive. Women who do this report feeling confident going into their pregnancies. They chose their provider without the pressure of needing one right away. You should be seen earlier than 9 weeks if

- you are unable to keep down fluids or food

- you need help establishing a good nutritional regimen

- you have other physical or psychological health issues that may complicate the pregnancy

- you will feel better establishing an early relationship with your provider

- you have any reason to suspect a miscarriage (excessive bleeding with large clots being passed)

- you suspect that something else is wrong (a woman's intuition that something is not right is usually the first symptom she will get—act upon this knowledge and consult a provider)

Should I keep my current ob-gyn?

PREGNANCY CARE IS DIFFERENT than gynecological care. Yet women often move without questioning from well-woman care to pregnancy care with the same provider. It is important to be aware that the physician you see may not be able to offer you a complete range of settings for your birth. This is because some providers only do hospital births in certain hospitals, while others only do homebirths or birth center births. It's great to love your gynecologist. But when you walk into a hospital for your birth, you are no longer protected by the good judgment and intentions of that provider. You are under the protocols of the hospital. These protocols are often written by attorneys whose job it is to protect their employer from legal action. They have no relevance to your right to choose how to birth and which sorts of technologies to use. While we support women who choose to birth in a hospital and believe that women should give birth wherever they feel safe, this choice should be a purposeful decision that you make, not the default you stumble into.

If we could pick one item that women struggle with most, it is this one: getting to the eighth month of pregnancy and suddenly realizing that they do not want to birth in the hospital. It is very stressful to search for homebirth care in the eleventh hour. We advise women to work backward, envisioning the kind of birth experience that they want and then finding a provider who will support them in this great adventure and be a partner with them on their journey. In this relationship, you hold the power. You are a consumer with consumer rights. You should set the tone and pitch of your experience, and define what matters most to you. Your provider should support, guide, and promote the path that you choose.

I want an out-of-hospital birth. Which providers give me this option?

THERE ARE MANY PRACTITIONERS to choose from if you want to give birth at home or in a birth center. It is your job to gain a good understanding of the training, education, and experience of any provider you work with. It is fairly easy to generate a list of local providers (to consider interviewing) just by making some phone calls or checking online. Here are some of your options:

Direct-Entry Midwife (DEM)

A DEM HAS A wide range of training and experience that lends to her abilities and safety in practice. She may or may not have attended midwifery school but will have acted as a midwife's apprentice for a period of one to three years or longer. She may or may not have credentials or a license to practice midwifery issued by her state. These credentials may not even be available in her state. To understand who she is and how she practices, you will need to interview her and speak with other women she has worked with. DEMs can be as qualified as any credentialed, licensed midwife. These women are trained on the front lines and often focus on self-directed learning within the context of a clinical experience.

Note: *DEMs work with normal healthy birthing mothers and attend homebirths. They are typically paid in cash.*

Certified Professional Midwife (CPM)

A CPM IS A midwife who is credentialed by the North American Registry of Midwives (NARM). The NARM verifies that her education and skills are of a certain standard of competency. CPMs have a minimum of three years of midwifery-based education or its equivalent and at least one year of apprenticeship with a qualified midwife. In some states, a CPM qualifies a midwife for licensure while in others she must pass additional exams and take additional trainings.

Note: *CPMs will typically work with healthy birthing mothers and attend homebirths or freestanding birth center births. CPMs may be cash-pay or accept insurance, depending on the rules of the state in which they practice.*

Licensed Midwife (LM)

A LICENSED MIDWIFE IS normally a CPM who has applied for and undergone the testing or other requirements of her state in order to practice midwifery there.

Note: *LMs will typically work with healthy birthing mothers and attend homebirths or births at freestanding birth centers. LMs typically accept insurance, although this depends on the rules of their particular state. Currently, twenty-three states license midwives.*

Certified Nurse-Midwife (CNM)

A CNM IS A registered nurse (RN) who has a master's degree in midwifery. Because she is credentialed to work in a hospital, she can often provide care for a woman who is high risk and therefore not considered a good fit for a homebirth. CNMs also work with women who want midwifery care with a hospital birth.

Note: *Many CNMs will work with birthing women at their homes or in the hospital setting, although some do not attend homebirths either because they choose not to or because they are not allowed to due to malpractice insurance regulations. Some attend births in freestanding birth centers. This varies from state to state. CNMs typically accept insurance.*

Physicians: Chiropractic, Family Practice, Naturopathic, Obstetric, and Osteopathic Doctors

A CHIROPRACTOR, NATUROPATH, OR osteopathic physician may have additional training in homebirth. These practitioners work with healthy birthing mothers in their homes or in freestanding birth centers. There are obstetricians and family practice MDs who do homebirths in certain communities.

So what is midwifery care?

MIDWIFERY IS BOUND BY two philosophies: the midwifery model of care and shared decision making. The official midwives model of care document was written in 1996 by several midwifery associations and the lay group Citizens for Midwifery. It was designed to provide shared language about the kind of care midwives offer. This model of care includes a midwife's obligation to monitor the physical, psychological, and social well-being of the mother and baby in a holistic way.

Midwives view clinical information in the context of a woman's life and unique self. Midwives provide individualized education, counseling, and care. They believe that a woman is capable of gathering information and making a decision that is right for her and her baby. Midwifery care encourages a woman and her partner to take responsibility for all decision making, while the midwife provides tools and resources to assist them in this process.

Many midwives offer continuity of care and provide prenatal, birth, and postpartum support for their clients as opposed to practicing in large groups where relationships are harder to form. The midwife minimizes use of technology without compromising safety. She uses her hands and mind, her heart and knowledge, to observe and draw conclusions about the health of a woman's pregnancy and birth. Midwives use blood pressure monitoring devices, stethoscopes, or Dopplers to listen to the baby, and lab testing as necessary to monitor the health of the mother and baby.

Shared decision making is a core value of midwifery care. This process provides midwives and parents the knowledge that all decisions made regarding care during the prenatal, birth, and postpartum periods are made together. It is the midwife's responsibility to ensure that educated decision making is accomplished, through the sharing of evidence-based research and experience. It is the parent's role to actually decide upon a course of care.

How do I hire a provider?

IT'S TIME TO PUT on your business hat! The first step in hiring a midwife is to develop a job description. Sit with your significant other or trusted friend and make an outline of the kind of person, attention, and care you want during your pregnancy. Don't limit yourself—this is your chance to explore your ideal experience and name the things that are important to you.

After you have generated a clear idea of what you want, hit the streets and get to know some providers. We recommend starting with three. Interview them. You may find the perfect fit, or at the very least have a much better idea of what you are looking for. Many midwives offer "meet and greets." These are free sessions that give you the opportunity to get to know them, to learn about the kind of practice philosophy they have, and to ask questions.

Most of all, you want someone you can really connect with. This organic bond is one that many mothers recall with fondness when discussing their pregnancy and birth.

What questions should I ask when I interview providers?

WE HAVE PROVIDED A comprehensive list of questions to consider asking a midwife in Appendix A. However, a successful relationship feels good, and you will recognize that feeling.

How will I know if I've found the right fit?

THE DECISION OF WHO you choose to work with is often made with the heart more than with the head. Ask yourself some questions:

- Do you feel safe with this midwife?
- Do you feel that decision making is shared and that you are not pressured to agree with her?
- Does your midwife encourage you to bring questions to each appointment and does she give you thorough answers that include additional resources for you to explore?
- Are you pleased with the care she is providing?

Trust your inner voice to tell you, "She's the one" or "Keep looking." Even as you get further along in your pregnancy, it is never too late to transfer into another practice if you're not comfortable with your provider. We know lots of moms who switched providers at 37, 38, and even 39 weeks of pregnancy. They often report that it feels like they are breaking up with a boyfriend in high school—it's hard but they know they have done the right thing and are happy to be moving on.

Hopefully with the tools provided here, you will find the perfect fit at the start of your pregnancy and enjoy a long-term relationship with a provider who is just right for you!

Prenatal Nutrition

What should I be eating during the first days and weeks of pregnancy?

YOUR NUTRITION IS AN accumulation of what you've been putting in your body over the course of a lifetime. Hopefully you have been eating a balanced diet full of green leafy vegetables and protein sources prior to conception. If you have not, there is great news: it's not too late to get on track! Adjusting your diet during pregnancy can profoundly improve your health as well as that of your baby. What you put in your body matters. Your baby thrives because of the health of your placenta, and she faces more challenges when that placenta is missing key nutritional components. Consider the idea that every bite you take can be packed with the nutrition needed to grow that placenta and nourish your baby. This awareness can help inspire meaningful nutritional choices.

There are many diets designed for pregnant women, but mothers today are busy with families and/or careers, and it's generally not realistic to expect them to follow a specific diet all day long for ten months. More importantly, developing good eating inclinations during pregnancy can lead to a lifetime of health and well-being. The practice seems to last longer if the choices become intuitive and not just something on a list to follow. It is very profound for us to see a woman come in for a visit with dull-looking skin and a sense of fatigue, help her adjust her diet, and see her return in a week or two looking bright-skinned and energetic. When it comes to pregnancy, it just feels better to eat well. This tends to help moms make choices that are right for their babies and themselves.

So here's the deal. We'll keep it simple and to the point. Sugar doesn't work for you or your baby. Processed, packaged foods should be the low man on the totem pole. If you're having some crackers with your lunch of green leafy veggies and salmon, great! If you're munching on crackers between meals, you are blocking your best energy.

The enemy of the midwife is not hospital birth. The enemy of the midwife is the pretzel. For some reason, pretzels are commonly thought of as the "healthy" alternative to potato chips. They aren't. They, and other highly processed carbohydrates, are just like a candy bar to your body. They can push many women from states of health that are slightly concerning straight into gestational diabetes.

If a woman has high blood sugar levels, it will affect the way she can nourish her baby. It also weakens her tissue integrity, so she tends to tear and bleed a lot more at the time of birth and be much harder to suture. Her baby may need nutritional support after birth as it struggles to balance sugar levels in its own body without the resources it had while en utero. And that is the part you can see—what you can't see but what you should know, is that while a mother is carrying a baby and eating too many sugar and white-flour–based products, the baby's body is working overtime to compensate for her choices. Before they're even born, babies' organs can be stressed.

The trick is balancing what goes in so that you get good amounts of proteins, carbs, vegetables, and fruits—they all work together to create a healthy you. Just to be clear, because we've been misunderstood before: "balance" does not mean ordering a salad with your pizza or double bacon cheeseburger. We are referring specifically to eating a variety of food from natural, unprocessed sources so that your taste buds and your body will be happy. Eating small meals regularly throughout the day can help keep blood sugar levels and nausea in check.

We have included a lot of detailed nutrition advice in chapter nine, where we discuss gestational diabetes. Although it may seem odd to be directed toward information on a disease you probably don't have, we suggest that all mothers eat as if they want to avoid the most common disease caused by poor nutritional choices. Meanwhile, here's a short list of great foods that will nourish your body while giving the most benefit to your baby:

- fish, chicken, beef, eggs
- green leafy vegetables
- colorful vegetables
- fresh fruits
- nuts, seeds, and legumes
- dark chocolate in moderation

What else should I be doing at this time?

OUR FIRST ANSWER IS a question back to you: What do you feel like doing? Take note of when your energy is at its strongest and what time of day it feels like you need to rest. You know your body best, and learning to follow its cues is one enduring gift of pregnancy. We have times in our monthly and daily cycles when we feel extroverted and creative as well as times when we need quiet reflection. Our babies experience this with us during pregnancy as the hormones that create these emotions cross the placenta.

- CONSIDER YOUR STRESS: Mamas teach their babies about honoring their bodies and reducing tension from the beginning of pregnancy. When times are tough, spend a few minutes to soothe and remind yourself and your baby that although there is stress, you are capable of recovering and moving forward. While we hope that all babies are conceived, baked, and then birthed in love, we know that reality can be a bit different! We also know that your child's life will include moments that are painful or stressful and they will recall the sensation of recovering from the patterning that you establish now. So consider your stress a gift that allows you to teach your baby that the world is a forgiving place where we can recover, heal, and move forward.

- TAKE THE TIME TO REALLY EXPERIENCE JOY EACH DAY: Make a short list of the activities that feed your soul. Choose some activities that can be accomplished easily and others that require more planning. Each morning when you get dressed, take a look at the list and pick something to engage in. Feeling joy releases chemicals into your body that soothe and nourish you and your baby.

- MOVE! Research has shown time and time again that movement generates both physical and mental health. Turn on some music and dance it up—you can do this alone, with your children, girlfriends, or partner. Taking a five- to ten-minute walk after meals helps release hormones that will convert your food into energy in an effective way. Your heart also needs exercise. Over the course of your pregnancy, it will be responsible for pushing 50 percent more in blood volume through your body. Follow your body and find something that feels great. Swimming is a hugely popular activity, as is brisk walking. Whatever it is that moves you to move, do it regularly and for a minimum of thirty minutes per day.

- TAKE YOUR PRENATAL VITAMINS: Consult your midwife for the vitamins you should be taking in addition to the standard prenatal vitamin. Be sure to ask about vitamin B_6, B_{12}, and D_3, as well as whether you need extra iron.

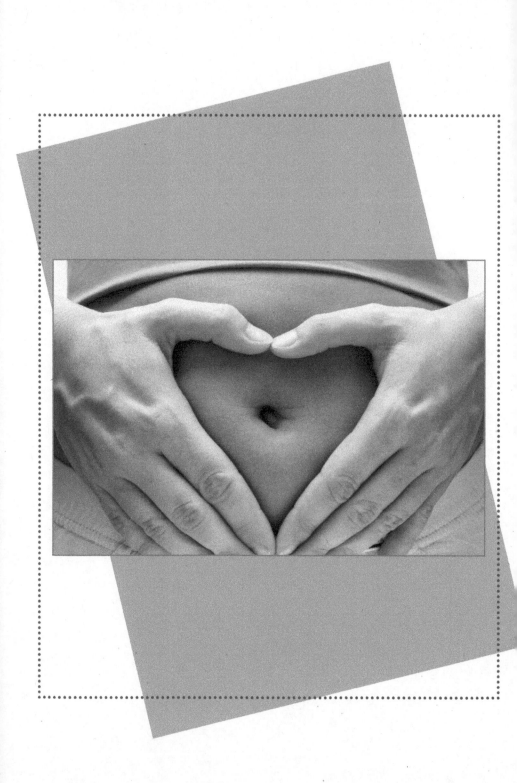

CHAPTER THREE

Prenatal Care with a Homebirth Midwife: More Than Just the Numbers

- The primary goal of prenatal care: establishing individualized norms
- Relationship development
- Welcome to your prenatal visit

MAMA SAYS

I would recommend a midwife one thousand times over. With a midwife, you get women-centered care that includes longer visits, a lower cost, and lots of education. I have read that midwifery care improves pregnancy outcomes, and I believe it!

My favorite part was feeling like I was visiting with a wise friend who had a wide range of knowledge and my best interests at heart. My least favorite part was the six-week postpartum visit, only because I hated saying good-bye!

My midwife made a difference in my life. She then went on to midwife my adult daughter and to make a huge impact in *her* life. I can never say enough about the impact midwifery care made on two different generations of my family.

—Kendra

The Primary Goal of Prenatal Care:
Establishing Individualized Norms

A WOMAN IS A unique human being, with more in her heart and in her life than can possibly be summarized on a medical chart or explained by mere statistics. That is why the primary goal of prenatal care is establishing individual norms—what is normal for you.

"Establishing individual norms" sounds like a contradiction in terms! What are individual norms and why are they important in pregnancy?

"INDIVIDUAL NORMS" IS A holistic mind-set that forms the foundation of midwifery care. When you come to a midwife for prenatal care, you bring your whole life with you. Your history, environment, support systems, stressors, nutrition, work, and play are all pieces of the big picture that is you.

You are more than a collection of numbers, statistics, and averages. That is why within a midwife's practice, norms are considered important but not the end-all. What is more important is determining *your* norms—recognizing what is "just right" for you.

Once we have established your individual normals, then together we can make a care plan for your pregnancy. We do this through the lens of what standardized norms tell us, but also by looking at who you are in the context of your whole life.

How can norms, which are standard or average by nature, possibly be individualized?

INDIVIDUALIZED NORMS ARE ESTABLISHED by looking at your medical history and comparing it to averages for any given issue. Norms help the medical profession provide standards of care and practice, but can be too limiting. For example, yours may be considered a high-risk pregnancy merely because of your age. The midwife determines if this average applies to you. Who knows? You may be more fit than the typical woman half your age. Given your overall health and lifestyle, you may be just as likely to birth at home with no complications as a much younger woman—and should be allowed to do so!

Why are individualized norms important?

AT YOUR INITIAL VISIT, a series of blood draws, tests, measurements, and a complete physical exam are all done to establish your baseline. Part of establishing what is normal for you includes sharing personal information regarding your physical, emotional, and spiritual health. The more 411, the better! Nothing is too small or unimportant, medically, psychologically, socially, or otherwise. At your first visit, consider sharing with your midwife pre-pregnancy lab work, medical records, and therapist's or spiritual advisor's notes.

There will be some areas your midwife will want to tweak through the use of supplements and nutrition, or even medication. This allows her to customize her expectations and to care for your body and your baby in a way that is just right for you.

Can you provide me with examples of how individualized norms may affect a pregnancy?

FIRST, TIMELY AND OPEN sharing of your information sets the tone for an open and honest relationship with your midwife. The ball is truly in your court—your midwife will ask for information but it is yours to share: your information, your choice, your responsibility. The information you bring, combined with the facts gathered through tests and lab work, allows the midwife to create a very personalized level of care. She will cater the information she shares with you—the way she presents options and even the options themselves—based on what she knows about you.

Let's say you don't like to drink water (a surprisingly common occurrence). Your midwife will incorporate that knowledge into your nutrition plan. As noted earlier, in pregnancy your blood volume increases by around 50 percent. Blood volume is composed of protein, salt, and water. If you don't put enough protein, salt, and water into your body, it will take what it needs from other systems to accommodate the requirements. Telling your midwife that you have a hard time drinking water gives her the opportunity to make sure that your hydration needs are met in a different way. Or consider this example of a mom neglecting to mention part of her medical history:

> I had a client who dilated extremely slowly over the course of four days. We tried everything: every position, every homeopathic remedy, and every visualization known to womankind. Nothing helped. Eventually the mom and baby became clinically exhausted, and we transferred to the hospital, where the baby was delivered by cesarean section. Later, the mother divulged that she had had three procedures on her cervix. These procedures can cause a build-up of scar tissue on the cervix. Unfortunately, she never mentioned it during any of the prenatal visits or while in labor. If I had known, the mom could have been treated prenatally with evening primrose oil or during labor by manually breaking up the scar tissue. Because this client's condition only came out after the cesarean, I missed the opportunity to provide individualized care.
>
> —Joanne (midwife)

We believe each woman should be looked at as a whole and vital member of her family, her community, and society. If she has medical risks, and a midwife looks at these in the context of her entire life, the midwife is more likely to have a positive influence on her and her baby's health. The midwifery model of care provides a platform for this holistic practice.

Relationship Development

What is "relationship development" and why is it listed as one of the midwife's goals for prenatal care?

THIS IS A FAVORITE topic among homebirth midwives. We like to think of our jobs as getting paid to fall in love with people over and over again. Parents report feelings of being heard, understood, and felt within the context of this care. Trust develops and builds as personal stories, history, and fears are shared with a loving midwife. Everything we humans do, we do best within the context of relationships. This includes putting the clinical picture of your pregnancy in its proper context. That baby you'll soon be holding in your arms will develop her sense of self and understanding of the world entirely within her relationship with you. Midwives take this model and run with it, providing the space, time, and open-hearted stance as a platform for mothers to thrive in their pregnancy and early parenting.

What is the current medical model of care?

WITH RARE EXCEPTION, THE standard model for prenatal care is all about numbers. Weight, fundal growth, blood pressure, fetal heart tones, vaginal exams, and lab results are all measured against the number of weeks of gestation and any risks that a mother presents with. A clinical picture emerges within about seven to fifteen minutes of face time with a nurse practitioner or OB. You receive handouts that cover relevant topics. The visits are usually pleasant enough, and most mothers enjoy hearing the tiny heart beating from within. Yet many mothers report feelings of anxiety and fear around these visits, largely because they know the person they are working with even for those short periods of time will likely not attend the birth.

This model of care is only expanding. Specialized "hospitalists" who do nothing but deliver babies full time and OBs who do only prenatal care are not somewhere down the road: the future is here. We believe that there are many obstetricians who go into the field with every intention of working with women in meaningful ways. However, the reality of the American medical system has squashed these caring folks and their ideas right down the medical waste disposal chute and into the incinerator.

Your Choices Matter

Here's something radical: having a live mother and baby *and* having a mind-blowing relationship with your provider are not mutually exclusive. It is all achievable and it is achievable because midwives view you holistically. A lot happens between the time of conception and diapers, and it all matters. It will affect you. It will change you. It will propel you into motherhood in a profound way and can leave you with feelings of power, health, and peace, or it may leave you with feelings of anxiety, fear, and even trauma. What kind of emotional context do you want as you become a new mother? What kind of new mother do you aim to be? Think about these questions first, and then start building your prenatal care to lead yourself down the road that ends with you—the kind of new mother you intend to become in the kind of health you strive to have.

Midwives believe deeply that all of the processes involved in becoming pregnant, being pregnant, and getting unpregnant are important. You are more than a vessel for an unborn child. You are a whole woman and you deserve prenatal care that honors this.

The medical model of care seems like it will keep me and my baby safe. Do I need all this relationship stuff?

IN A NUTSHELL, WITHOUT relationships we suffer in our work. Doctors are not immune to this and many find themselves feeling burned out by overloaded schedules with women they don't really know. They have a heavy emotional workload as they enter a small exam room, quickly assess the state of the woman who is there, and meet her where she is emotionally. This process is easier if a relationship is established. When you see a friend feeling enthusiastic, upset, or relaxed, it is quick business to meet their emotional state and interact with them in a meaningful way. But the psychological toll of doing this many times a day with people one doesn't know is quite profound and has been shown to cause burnout in all service-related industries.[1] Research on burnout among doctors has shown that when they see their patients as objects and not real people with whole lives, their clinical skills suffer. They feel they are on autopilot and do not find meaning in their work. Forget all of the medical interventions offered at a typical hospital birth and the questions easily built up around them. Is this the relationship you want with your care provider? Midwives are certainly not above this slip into the depths of overscheduled, undernourished work lives. When you write your list of questions to ask a potential provider, just add this one to your list: "Do you feel burned out by your work and how do you handle it if you do?"

Okay, my provider's not perfect. Can't I fill in the gaps on my own?

MOTHERS SURF THE WEB at ungodly hours and read lots of books to fill in the blanks left by short visits with a provider who doesn't really know her. Additionally we women lack the mother/sister wisdom we once thrived upon and turn to online forums for these connections. How big is your baby this month? What systems are developed? What food should you eat for optimal nutrition? What sensations are normal and which should be reported? Truly, the list goes on and on. We are all for reading books and gathering facts. We are research junkies ourselves. Yet the quantity of conflicting information online and in print will have a mother spinning in circles in less time than it takes to say "Google." Women who try to discuss studies with their doctors are often seen as challenging and difficult patients, rather than educated, curious, and insightful women. Dr. Donald Winnicott, a protégé of Freud, had concerns regarding the volume of pamphlets being handed out to new mothers and the effect this may have on a woman's belief in herself as capable and knowing. We look to his wise words, spoken way back in the 1940s and '50s regarding the vast quantity of reading material a new mother is drowned in: "If she does what she is told, she has to go on doing what she is told, and to improve she can only choose somebody better to tell her what to do. But if she is feeling free to act in the way that comes naturally to her, she grows in her job."[2]

Today, instead of a few pamphlets, we have Amazon.com. A mother will find nearly 20,000 books if she searches the word "pregnancy," 45,000 if she searches the word "birth," and more than 57,000 if she searches the word "parenting." The remedy for this is to sit quietly and explore what you know. Develop a relationship with a trusted provider who will guide you to a few hand-selected resources that fit your interests and needs. And most importantly, approach these people and the information you come across with the knowledge that you are your own best expert. A midwife is a member of your team. You are the coach, the captain, and the referee. We are your cheerleaders, your water-girls, and your pregame strategists.

With few exceptions, midwives do not view prenatal care as a time to put information into your head, but as a process of exposing what you already know to be true. They work with you to develop and expand that knowledge base. Along the way, they may recommend some great Web sites and books but only to backfill your knowledge with research or options.

How is this accomplished over the course of my prenatal care?

THE SIMPLE ANSWER IS the one remedy midwives prescribe the most: a tincture of time. Your initial visit with your midwife may be between one and two hours long. You'll laugh, you'll have fun, and you'll share your stories and hear hers (or his!). You'll do such fabulous things as learn how to read the results of urine tests and interpret your blood pressure readings. We will measure and celebrate your growth. You will receive a complete physical exam wearing your own clothing and not a drafty gown. Depending upon the laws of your state (or province for our Canuck friends), your blood will be drawn and sent off to the lab for analysis. We love this visit. It's great getting to know a new person and establishing the foundation for what we trust will grow to be a deep and meaningful relationship. By the end of the visit, we will already be integrating hard numbers with what we hear and learn from you. What midwives and the mothers who hire them know, is that somewhere in the midst of sharing this time together, a relationship begins to grow.

Welcome to Your Prenatal Visit

Where will my prenatal visit take place?

MANY MIDWIVES HAVE THEIR own offices, but others will do some or all of your prenatal visits in your home. The convenience factor is high for home-based care, but some women find the office atmosphere more conducive to intimate discussions. Sometimes it's difficult to talk about hemorrhoids when you can hear Sponge Bob yammering about crabby patties in the living room.

So what happens at each prenatal visit?

THE FIRST THING MOTHERS do at each office visit with either a midwife or an OB is urinate into a small cup. This is tested for traces of protein and glucose, which can be harbingers of two serious complications: preeclampsia and gestational diabetes. In the obstetrician's office, you hand off the cup to a medical assistant, who whisks it away, never to be seen again. If there are abnormal results, your doctor will share them with you and create a plan to address the issues.

However, as we mentioned earlier, your midwife will teach you to test your own urine. She will show you exactly how to dip the test strip into the sample and interpret the results. It's not rocket science, nor is the knowledge sacred. You don't need to be a professional to match colors on a stick. This may seem like a relatively small thing, but you see what we're getting at: mothers are viewed as intelligent and capable and are expected to take an active role in their care on many levels, at all times.

After you tell your midwife your results, you can settle in for a nice, long chat. The average homebirth midwife's appointment lasts between thirty and sixty minutes and should never feel rushed. Normal topics of conversation include what you have felt or wondered about since your last visit, how your work and home life are coming along, your nutrition, exercise, and sleep, and, of course, your baby. Your questions will be answered fully and completely. If there are any tests or other procedures coming up, you will be given the pros and cons of each so that you can make informed decisions about your care.

As you get closer to your birth, you will start to imagine what that will look and feel like. The conversation shifts to the physiology of your bones, muscles, and skin, as well as the philosophy and psychology of your ideal birth. You may have questions about what to have on hand or when to call. If you're not satisfied with the answers, ask again. Do what it takes to get clarity on the issues that are important to you. Your midwife will expect this model for discussions and decision making. Some women, though, find these kinds of discussions almost overwhelming at first. For example,

Our questions were always addressed immediately and answered completely. Our midwives weren't shy about expressing their opinions about most things. When I needed to make a choice, they gave me the pros and cons and left the decision in my hands. At first, I felt nervous that I was given so much "freedom," but I also knew that that is exactly how it should be. I had no conditions or problems in my pregnancy, was healthy and strong, and ready to deliver at home.

There was no need to fuss over me or push anything on me. I was responsible for my own birth experience. Having this much responsibility was tough at times, but it also allowed me to learn and grow and really get into it. Nine months later, this led to a wonderful birth experience.

—Kelli

What kinds of clinical work do midwives do at prenatal visits?

MIDWIVES ARE QUITE LITERALLY hands-on in their care. We do a variety of checks that are clinical in nature to track your norms, growth, and changes.

Your blood pressure will be taken at each visit during pregnancy to monitor for any major changes, as your blood volume increases by 50 percent and the cardiovascular system works overtime to compensate for this. Your blood pressure is one indicator of how well your body handles these demands. Your midwife should always tell you the exact reading. For most women this is merely one piece of the whole picture of your pregnancy. If there are problems, midwives usually look to your nutrition and exercise regimen for solutions. This is usually the time the midwife will ask you how your swelling is and she may take a peek at your ankles and fingers. Significant swelling is a meaningful symptom, and in conjunction with high blood pressure indicates the need for testing to determine the possible onset of preeclampsia. As with all medical issues, if it cannot be solved in the context of midwifery care, you will be referred to a specialist for further evaluation and treatment.

A little trick we have discovered is that eating one raw cucumber per day has significant health benefits: the trace minerals and vitamins inside a cucumber combine to reduce swelling and lower blood pressure. They are good for the teeth and gums and add luster to your fingernails. In pregnancy, an apple a day keeps the heartburn away and a cucumber a day keeps the doctor away!

Palpating bellies is one of our greatest joys, and sadly, this is becoming a lost art in many birthing circles. We use this touch as a way to communicate with the unborn baby, to let him know he is wanted, loved, and that the world will be a better place when he takes his place in it. There is no ESP or magic involved; we just choose to talk out loud to the baby as we are assessing his position. We talk to them in great earnestness about not kicking your bladder, what a great mom you are, or how awesome it is that they've chosen to reside with their head in your pelvic outlet instead of in your ribs. We follow the same pattern each time we check your baby's position. Is the back on the left or the right? Is the head or buttocks heading straight into the pelvis? Approximately how big is this baby? One midwife we know draws a picture of the baby on the mother's belly, showing exactly where the baby is sitting that day. Ask your midwife to show you how to palpate your own belly. It's even more fun to play with your baby when you know which part you are touching!

The final piece of this clinical side to your visit is a fundal-height check. Your midwife will measure, in centimeters, the distance between the top of your pelvis at your pubic joint and the top of your uterus. After 20 weeks, this measurement should correspond roughly to the number of weeks pregnant you are. A 36-centimeter belly usually indicates a baby that has been gestating for 36 weeks. The trend is more important than the actual number and can show if the baby is growing steadily and in a predictable way. If there is any question about your baby's growth, checking up on your baby via ultrasound is an option.

Some midwives offer additional to-dos at prenatal visits. Each of us adds our own spice and style to a typical visit, but it usually starts and ends with warm words of encouragement and a hug.

What is the typical schedule for prenatal visits?

ROUTINE OBSTETRICAL AND MIDWIFERY care follow roughly the same schedule. You will see your midwife once per month for the first 30 to 32 weeks, then twice per month until 36 weeks, and then once per week for the final 4 weeks. Most women look forward to the weekly check-ins at the end for the great pep talks and planning and celebration of the coming birth. If you get past 40 weeks of gestation, your midwife may want to see you more often and will ask you to keep a closer eye on your baby.

I'm sorry, did you just say past 40 weeks?!?

AH, YES. LET'S TAKE some time to discuss this issue, commonly re-ferred to as post dates. It is a fact that the majority of healthy pregnan-cies take just a wee bit longer than the textbook-suggested 40 weeks. The average first-time mother goes eight days past her "due date." Ba-bies have absolutely no concept of the Julian calendar, and live only in that time outside of time, that holy space that the Greeks call *kairos*. This time bears no relation to the normal, everyday time we keep track of on our watches and calendars, called *chronos*. *Kairos* is that non-linear, nonrational place where there is no forward or backward, only now. It's why your grandmother can speak about her late husband as if he is just running an errand. It's why you and your best friend from high school can pick up exactly where you left off, even though you lost contact more than ten years ago. *Kairos* is very real and an element of pregnancy that may not be discussed enough. Mothers, fathers, and birth workers reflecting upon a birth will often note that "it felt as though time had no meaning and was suspended." Consider *chronos* a useful tool that humans invented as a way to make plans, impose our will and control on the universe, and sell more cute kitchen calendars. When it comes to pregnancy, you are both suspended in *kairos* and bound by *chronos*.

It's pretty hard to get a grip on the fact that you are actually at the intersection of both kinds of time. Your head is living in *chronos* and wants so much to meet your baby. And your body, on a very concrete cellular and chemical level, is living with your baby in *kairos*. The birth is only the last day of your pregnancy. Until this point, you have been doing beautifully for all of the minutes, hours, weeks, and months nurturing and caring for your baby. This pregnancy will end when the time is right for your baby to be born. One "overdue" mother sent this e-mail update to her midwife as she sailed right past that 40-week mark:

> Hello,
>
> Thanks so much for your e-mail yesterday and for checking on us today.
>
> Your words reminded me of many things that I know are important and that I've been trying to keep in mind during this pregnancy. I'm not in control. The medical community is not. Even my pro-natural-birth pals are not. For a few minutes, when someone asked me why I was still pregnant, I felt sort of stupid and as though I'd missed some important body of knowledge.
>
> But you reminded me that I'm not stupid—I'm trying to go about this in yet another way.
>
> On faith. Trying to jump-start the process is still trying to control it.
>
> Today I read something written by a French priest in the mid-1800s. "Joy is a dilation and an exaltation of the soul." Joy and dilation together! Hurray!
>
> So I'm contentedly hanging out in *kairos*. I'm uncomfortable, but I'm not desperate or anxious. I'm contemplating what kind of wardrobe changes I'd need to make in case I really do stay this shape forever. Because in *kairos*, that is a possibility.
>
> I know progress is still being made. I woke up early this morning with my thighs aching from my hip sockets to my knees. The baby feels even lower and my contractions are taking on a new quality. My digestion is still very regular, and not yet "diarrears" (which is what one of my great uncles called it.

He also cooked food in a "formicawave.") No bloody show, no mucus plug.
Love,
Tiff

Tiffany had her baby 4 days after she sent this e-mail. If you, too, are post dates, check in with your baby (ten movements per hour is normal) and your body. Your midwife can refer you for non-stress tests that take a look at the baby's well-being by assessing his heart rate and reaction to any contractions you may be having. Use what you feel and what you know and listen to whatever that little voice in your head is telling you—discussing issues with your midwife as they come up is as vitally important in these last days of your pregnancy as it was in your first. For more information on post dates pregnancy, please read After the Due Date in chapter ten.

You didn't mention getting weighed at my appointments. Why not?

IT IS A RARE American woman who doesn't carry some emotional baggage surrounding her weight. From moms who put us on diets before puberty to the out-of-control skinny models selling everything from cars to candy bars, we are bombarded every day of our life with conflicting, damaging messages. By the time we reach the childbearing years, our brains are swimming in expectation and fantasy regarding weight and appearance. We would be missing the mark to think that these messages lose their power in pregnancy, or that weighing a woman as part of her regular care may not bring up feelings of fear or painful memories.

My pregnancy with my first child was one of the most torturous experiences of my life. I am over six feet tall, and I am not a thin woman. My doctors blew up my "white-coat" syndrome into preeclampsia, in spite of good blood work and no real symptoms other than a higher baseline blood pressure. I was so nervous in the doctor's office that of course my baseline was going to be higher. I've dealt with doctors all my life who prejudge my health just by looking at me. The doctors pushed me into taking a very dangerous drug, despite the fact that my blood pressure was fine at home and at work. They pressured me into constant testing. I had six ultrasounds, and fifteen non-stress tests (NSTs). It was insane. During my last NST they told me they were going to induce my labor, or I would lose my baby. They actually promised I would have a dead baby. After a guilt-ridden induction process (a three-day sentence in labor and delivery), I promised myself that if I was to have another baby, I would do it my way.

I became pregnant a few years later. I had just lost my job, and we feared we would lose our home. The pregnancy couldn't have seemed to have come at a worse time. In spite of this, I had an indescribably wonderful experience.

We decided on a midwife. The prenatal care was very complete, yet unobtrusive with no unnecessary testing. I could do everything my way. We had long prenatal visits, where I was told I was a normal healthy woman, in spite of my size. I had no excessive poking or prodding. I was encouraged to continue to work out, and eat right, which I truly did. Even with all the external stress in my life at this time, I will never be able to thank my midwife enough for the joy I took out of my pregnancy. She believed me when I told her big does not necessarily equal sick, and my baby proves it.

—Jennifer

For some women, pregnancy is a wonderful time with regard to self-image; they make friends with their body, perhaps for the first time. They recognize and honor the intense work their body is doing, and do their very best to support it through nutrition, exercise, and lots of time for self-exploration. Birthing is almost always an experience of coming into physical and emotional power for women. For some mothers, this process starts with pregnancy and manifests through an uber-interest in and dedication to great nutrition, exercise, and self-care. These women's bodies grow babies that are just the right size for them. There is rarely an exception to this rule unless a mother interferes with the natural ratio by taking in too many calories or calories too light in nutrients.

> Food is the most intimate thing you can buy. . . . Unlike clothes and shoes that dress the outside, food goes into your body and builds who you become.
>
> —Ani Phyo

On the other hand, many women struggle with eating well, an eating disorder, or weight issues in general. They may feel inadequate because they think of themselves as too fat or too thin to meet society's expectations. A woman who has dealt with eating disorders in the past may find that her current pregnancy weight gain triggers something deep within. Still others may struggle to balance food aversion, morning sickness, or cravings with what they know to be healthy, whole food choices. They either avoid the scale or obsess over it. These mothers need support, not a lecture. If this sounds familiar to you, talk it through with your midwife. Sometimes a referral to a dietician or nutritionist can be very helpful. These professionals can help you expand your food choices, while still giving enough calories to grow a healthy, thriving baby. What you don't need is condemnation and judgment, be it from your midwife, yourself, or anyone else in your life.

Significant or sudden weight gain or loss during pregnancy can be a window into issues that may merit medical attention. For this reason we have spent a lot of time finding the balance between providing supportive and nonthreatening care and monitoring the numbers. The options that work well are these:

- Women can weigh themselves at each visit and report the number on the scale.
- Women can register their own weight at their first clinic visit at 0. They are responsible for recalling their weight from visit to visit and giving us updates such as "plus 4 lbs," which we will note in their chart.

- Women can keep track of their own weight at home using a good scale and report back just as above with the amount they have gained.

- If this is a major sticking point for a woman, we will talk through the issues and come to an arrangement. Not wanting to step on a scale should not stop anyone from seeking midwifery care.

Nutrition is everything in the midwifery world; for healthy home-births we need the extra layer of protection that only a wellness-based lifestyle can provide. Mothers and the babies they grow almost always do better when the calories Mom consumes during pregnancy are loaded with nutrients. In our experience, homebirthing mothers know this. If you are struggling, you know it. If you are living the Hostess life, you know it. If you need help, talk to your midwife. The scale won't give you holistic knowledge, nutritional information, or pep talks. Your midwife will, with a genuine smile on her face and an understanding for the hard work of taking the time to take care of yourself.

Samantha found that with just a little bit of tweaking her already healthy diet, she was able to improve the health of her pregnancy:

My first two births were in the hospital. I was induced with both at 39 weeks and they both weighed 7 lbs 12 oz. Both births were good but we really felt led to have our third at home. I ate as I did with my first two pregnancies; on the healthy end of the standard American diet. We did my one-hour glucose test and it came back just outside of the normal range so I decided to do the three-hour test. What a horrible experience. I don't have any problem getting my blood drawn but by the second blood draw, I was very woozy and passed out. I had to spend the rest of the time on the bed in the office. Two of the results came back fine and only one was high, indicating that I did not have gestational diabetes. I went on to eat the same way, indulging in things like ice cream four or five nights a week. I was pregnant and not gaining too much weight, so why not?

This baby came three days after my due date and the labor was normal. The head was crowning and I knew with one more push I would have the head out and then meet my baby. As it turns out, one push brought out the eyebrows, next the eyes, the next the nose, and finally the rest of the head. That was not what I expected. Then the shoulders got stuck. I now know this is called shoulder dystocia. I tried pushing while the midwife tried to free the shoulder. They told me to get on my hands and knees, hoping it would open up my pelvis. Somehow my husband flipped me over. On my hands and knees, the midwife continued to help the baby until I delivered my girl. She weighed 10 lbs, 11 oz. We had no idea she would be that big!! I had a postpartum hemorrhage and had to go to the hospital. We were happy to have had a homebirth, a healthy baby, and such amazing midwives. But I did not have the homebirth experience I had hoped for.

When we got pregnant with our fourth, I started to think about how people will tell you that each baby gets bigger. I wasn't expecting small babies as both my husband and I are tall, but clearly the last was a bit bigger than my body was made for. I thought back to my glucose tests and wondered if there really were diabetic-type issues. I knew I would never do the three-hour test again, and chose to work on my diet instead. At 28 weeks, I cut all refined sugars and flours. As a snack to satisfy the late-night ice cream craving, I had a yogurt parfait: whole milk yogurt sweetened with honey and then topped with strawberries, bananas, and almonds. I ate whole-wheat products and felt really good. I only gained 35 lbs. My son was born with no complications and was 10 lbs 2 oz. That half a pound made a big difference and there were no stuck shoulders this time. I'll never know if my previous baby got stuck because she was too big. There can certainly be shoulder dystocias with small babies. But I was determined to do everything in my power to help this baby come out. And I did. What an awesome birth.

I got pregnant again with baby number five. I had learned much more about nutrition and decided that I wanted to make even better choices. I knew this was especially important in the last trimester. At 28 weeks, I gave up all sweeteners and all grains. I ate meat, veggies, nuts, and fruit (Paleo diet). I never felt deprived—I felt fantastic. I let myself have something special but realized it only made me feel awful physically. My fifth baby arrived 10 days after his due date and weighed a measly 9 lbs. While that may seem like a big baby, he was nearly 2 pounds lighter than my third. There were no complications and I healed faster than after any of my other labors.

What you eat matters. As a matter of fact, it can be the difference between the lovely homebirth that you desire, and some very scary moments followed by a trip to the ER. I am so happy that I gave myself and my baby the food we deserved. Everyone was happier and healthier because of my good choices.

—Samantha

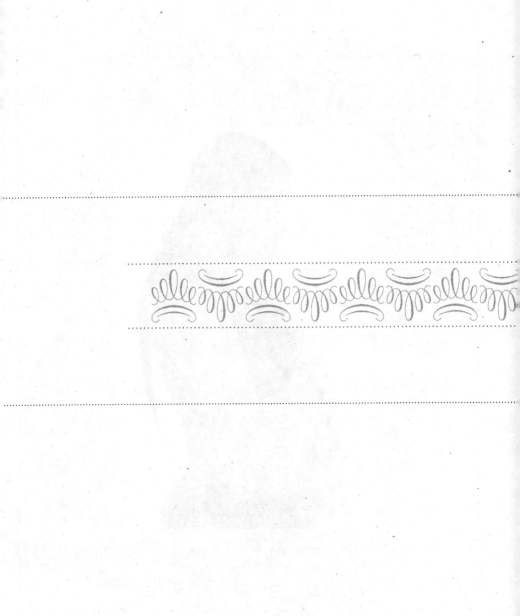

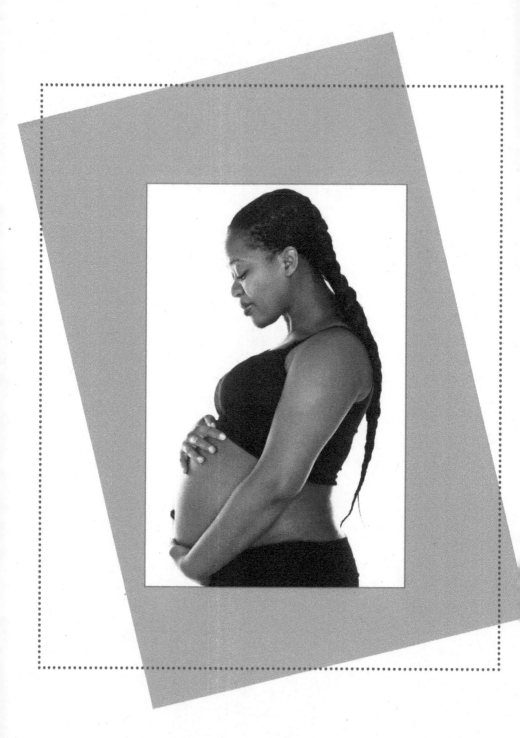

CHAPTER FOUR

Midwifery Care, Homebirth, and the Mother's Community

- Relationships
- Homebirth and family
- From co-workers to strangers, everyone wants a piece of me!
- Keeping calm and cared for

MAMA SAYS

My community is so supportive. They had questions about my homebirth, definitely, but once I explained everything, they all wanted to be a part of my birth. I felt like it was one big potluck supper. Everyone brought something wonderful to my birthing experience.

—Rosie

Relationships

BECAUSE YOUR PREGNANCY IS visible, others in your life will get caught up in your experiences or be drawn in by your expanding belly. Partners will join you in sharing the wonder and challenges of this time. Your parents will stare at you and wonder how their baby could possibly be having a baby. Strangers will suddenly be telling you their birth stories. You will be judged based upon the contents of your grocery cart. People in the elevator will touch you with no warning whatsoever. (Our favorite response to this very common experience was one mother who decided she would just rub people's bellies right back, staring at them and smiling in the same dreamy way they looked at her.)

The trick here is that you will be experiencing all of this through the physiological and psychological lens of pregnancy. It is fun, bizarre, exciting, terrifying, frustrating, and wonderful. You will meet your inner lioness, fiercely protective of your body and your baby. You will question if you are really ready for this, and wonder about the people you have surrounded yourself with and the choices you have made—there's so much to think about! You will face new challenges, and while you may stumble a bit on the way, you will conquer them.

Why does the rest of my life matter during prenatal care?

THE MIDWIFERY MODEL OF CARE encompasses your whole family, and to a certain extent your whole community. Expectant mothers are women first and pregnant second. We all have so many different facets of our identity. Let's take a holistic snapshot of who each mother might be: a partner, mother, daughter, breadwinner, girlfriend, carpool driver, board president, and sexual being. All of these aspects combine into a coherent whole and are honored under the midwifery model of care.

The road to baby isn't meant to be a simple one. It is meant to push and pull you, drop you on your rear, and send you flying. In a way, the ups and downs you face during your pregnancy prepare you for the challenges of parenting. Each part of you will be changed and challenged. It is a great time to embrace your sense of adventure. What an exciting ride!

When you are pregnant, your body and its demands are foremost in your mind. So how do you balance those demands, such as morning sickness, fatigue, and the need for extra calories, with the rest of your life? Sometimes just talking about your worries is helpful. Your midwife can help you make sense of the feelings you're experiencing. Midwifery care isn't just about your clinical picture. The pressures, successes, and challenges you face during your pregnancy *are* your pregnancy. And they all contribute to the vital information your midwife puts together about who you are. She will use all of it to help you experience your pregnancy in the most meaningful way possible. Amber learned this by accident when she struck up a conversation with a midwife at a local celebration:

I had started my pregnancy under the care of an obstetrician. I met a midwife at a community event and we started to talk about my pregnancy—I had some fears around whether or not I would be able to carry my baby to term. She gave me a rousing pep talk—detailing everything that was going right, talking about my baby as a partner in the pregnancy, and asking me all kinds of questions about my fears. She helped me see that spending the evenings reading Internet horror stories was causing me to sink further into my fear without offering any rest from my worries. She asked me to try an experiment—to forgo reading stories online for one week, substituting my Internet time with a five-minute walk outside, followed by something I loved to do. We talked about how the stories that I was reading online were from women who had difficulties that they were still processing. I understood for the first time that just because those women were still working through their trauma, it did not mean that all birthing stories ended terribly!

She also came over to my home later that day. She had offered to check the baby for us. I lay down on my bed and she asked permission to touch me (this was something new!). She then began to rub my belly and talk to the baby. My husband asked if she was doing some kind of low-tech ultrasound. She turned to me and asked if anyone had put their hands on my belly like this while I was pregnant. They had not. My appointments consisted of an ultrasound in the clinic room at each visit, rough hands pushing on my belly, and talking about what I should do next. Her gentle care, encouragement, and joy when the baby responded and kicked her hand made me cry. I didn't know that a provider could take all of my worries and relate them to my health and help me feel so positive and excited about my body and baby. It was magical.

Homebirth and Family

In what ways can I expect my relationship with my spouse or partner to change?

MANY COUPLES FIND THAT pregnancy deepens their relationships in ways they never imagined. We know this sounds like a cliché. It is, but it's also true. Watching a partner fall in love with a pregnant woman all over again is one of our greatest joys. Different couples have different challenges, but there is an opportunity for growth here that is unmatched by any other situation. Here, April, a first-time homebirther, describes her experience:

My relationship with my husband deepened during our pregnancy and subsequent homebirth. We had already been married for four years, but when we got pregnant it became an even greater partnership. We wanted to learn together how to take care of me, our unborn baby, and all that would follow on this journey. During the pregnancy we reached a new level of connectedness. He seemed to be in awe of the fact that I was growing our baby. Throughout my pregnancy, and especially after the birth, he would often say, "I'm so proud of you."

Honestly, there was a part of me that had questioned how deep our love was—not because of anything he did, but because of my own insecurities. The pregnancy (and birth for that matter) made me realize how connected and bonded we are as a couple.

The Midwife Says: Sometimes couples come to pregnancy already struggling, and the stress of a new baby can drive them even further apart. Other times, they may grow distant from one another during the pregnancy. We try to give our parents support for where they are at while providing opportunities for them to connect over their pregnancy and baby. While a midwife is not a therapist, you can expect her to be open-minded and really good at reflective listening. Both partners should be given the chance to express their feelings that have developed since the last appointment. Sometimes these feelings may be hard for the other partner to hear; those emotions are most likely the ones that really need to be shared. Don't be afraid to ask for a referral for couples counseling; it can really help as you make this adjustment.

What happens when one partner wants a homebirth and the other does not?

THIS IS A TOUGH one. Homebirth is the ultimate family affair, and it's important that everyone be on the same page. Ideally a couple

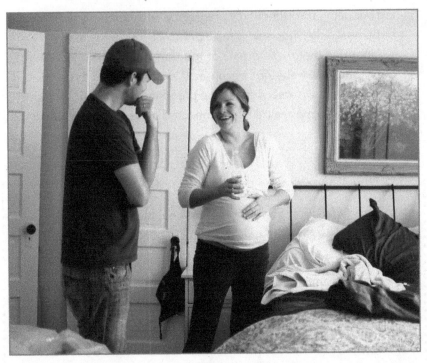

Relationships can and do grow, along with your belly.

decides together to have a homebirth, but that doesn't always happen. We have seen more than a few partners sit on the midwife's couch, their arms folded and lips pursed. A midwife can try to assuage any concerns with safety statistics, her training and experience, and the lifesaving equipment she keeps on hand. At the end of the day, it is not the midwife's role to talk anyone into having a homebirth. In fact, it is just the opposite. If you feel as if a midwife is glossing over risks, or painting too pretty a picture of homebirth, we respectfully suggest that you should interview other candidates. The midwifery model of care relies upon parent responsibility in decision-making, and should not include placing their ideals onto your birth. Most midwives will provide information about their practice and share their safety statistics. It will be important to your midwife that you are on the same page before you get too far along in your care.

If one of you desires a homebirth and the other does not, communication and patience are key. Some couples find the "Talking Stick

Method" of communication helpful. In many Native American cultures, the talking stick was used as a way to ensure that each person was able to speak to the council in a fair and meaningful way (this custom has many beautiful elements, which you can read about in the legends section of www.firstpeople.us). The following exercise is based on this practice.

To begin, one person holds an object, asks their partner a question, and then passes the object over. The partner then answers the question. While the speaker is talking, the listener simply listens without planning a response or rebuttal. He must concentrate on the speaker, acknowledging silently that whatever he is hearing is the partner's truth. For the speaker's part, she must not anticipate what the partner is going to say or be deliberately disrespectful. When the speaker is through, she passes the object to the listener, who then summarizes what he heard. If the speaker agrees that this is what was actually said, then the listener says his piece and the process continues. If the speaker disagrees, she gets back the object and has an opportunity to clarify.

Talking Stick Exercise Example

Parent A: (holding object) Can you tell me why a homebirth is so important to you? (passes object)

Parent B: (takes object) I am looking for a respectful, meaningful experience. I want a provider who really knows me, and you, and our family situation. I believe that birth is best when it is simple, and does not involve a lot of technology. I think our baby will be safer in our home. I'm looking forward to the challenge of birthing our baby naturally, and believe that pregnancy is not a medical condition. (passes object)

Parent A: (takes object) I hear that you do not believe you can get those things in a hospital. I also hear how important this is to you. (passes object)

Parent B: (takes object) That is true. (passes object)

Parent A: I am worried about the safety of you and our baby. I worry that something will go wrong, and there will be nothing I can do about it.

Parent B: I hear that you are worried about my and our baby's safety, and that you are worried that you won't know how to help me if something does go wrong. How would you feel about coming to my next prenatal appointment so that we can ask the midwife together about these issues? I feel safe and cared for with my midwife, and if you meet her, I think you will see why I feel this way.

And so the discussion continues.

This is not an issue that will be solved in a single talk. Both partners' wishes must be respected, if possible. If one person is completely uncomfortable after a lot of heartfelt communication, it may be worth seeking a compromise, such as a freestanding birthing center or a community hospital with a certified nurse midwife. Homebirth is not for everyone, and that is okay.

In what ways can I expect my relationship with my parents to change?

THE SHIFTING RELATIONSHIP WITH your parents is often one of the most gratifying experiences of pregnancy. As you grow into the role of mothering, you will naturally reflect upon your childhood and the parts of parenting that you want to carry forward or change. Women often ask their parents what it was like when their kids were young, seeing them from this all-new perspective of people who have been in the trenches and come out the other side. If there are unresolved issues from your childhood, this is a great time to address those. Your pregnancy hormones prime you for understanding, change, and growth.

Becoming a parent also requires you to define the role your parents will play in your new family's life. Open yourself to the wisdom both of your parents and yourself. Clear boundaries and open communication about your needs and expectations can raise your relationship with your parents to new levels.

If you anticipate that they will be very hands-on grandparents, be sure to take the time to teach them the ropes when it comes to all of the equipment you purchase. Unless you are a teenager, Diaper Genies weren't around when you were a kid and pins were required for fastening almost everything important. You may also feel more comfortable if your parents take an infant CPR class, available at your local Red Cross or fire station.

From Co-workers to Strangers, Everyone Wants a Piece of Me!

My co-workers have a lot to say about my condition and my plans for pregnancy and birth. I just want to do my job.

CO-WORKERS. THEY HOLD AN interesting spot in our community. Whether you seek out friendships at your job or spend your break time avoiding Loud Mouth Dan from IT, there is a pretty good chance that you spend more hours at work than with your family. Co-workers are the modern tribe, a group of people bound together by a common purpose for mutual benefit. And like all small villages, they can be constantly in your business.

Keep in mind, it is not your job to become the poster child for homebirth. When humans form groups, especially around a common goal, many folks assume that everyone thinks basically the same about everything. They know intellectually that this is not true, but on some basic level, we assume more sameness than difference. When someone embodies a different ideal, it can be threatening on a primal level.

You may be tempted to extoll the virtues of homebirth, quoting safety statistics and emergency plans, countering every argument with razor-sharp dialectics that would make Plato weep with joy. This can get extremely tiring, and you certainly have better things to do, like growing a person and getting that report out on time. If you are a budding homebirth activist, there are other venues to turn your passion into good.

Share the information you feel comfortable with, but if you find your time consumed by defending your choices, find a graceful exit to the conversation. It's best to have a couple of conversation stoppers ready to whip out. "Oh, thanks for your interest, but we've got everything covered." Or the more firm "We've already made this choice. It is not up for debate." And if all else fails, and the Water Cooler Menace doesn't respond to polite directness, you can always go to HR.

Pregnancy itself seems to be a constant topic of conversation regardless of birth location. The comments below came from real women, working in real jobs, with real co-workers. Izzy's co-worker apparently thinks she knows best, which is somewhat entertaining, but could be annoying:

Co-worker: How are you feeling?
Izzy: Fine.
Co-worker: No you don't. You're lying. Your back hurts and your body aches all over.
Izzy: Uh, okay. That's not true, but okay.

Lisa works in a predominantly male environment, with many people coming through her workplace every day. The sort of comment below is never acceptable in the workplace. Women are often blind-sided by such remarks and don't know how to respond. We have had many mothers tell us that a direct "Wow, that's really not appropriate" seems to work well.

> Mechanic: Wow, I almost didn't recognize you, you are getting really big!
> Lisa: Uh, thanks for that.
> Mechanic: No, don't get me wrong. It's great! I don't know what it is, but I find pregnant women incredibly sexy.
> Lisa: (awkward, confused look)
> Mechanic: Yeah, I never could figure it out, just something about them. . . .
> Lisa: (in a joking tone) Well, if you ever do figure it out, please don't feel obligated to tell me. You can keep that one to yourself.
>
> There were a few other guys around who kind of laughed it off when I laughed, but I mean, REALLY? Thanks for sexualizing my pregnant body at 7:00 a.m., co-worker!

Sometimes your co-workers may mean well, but simply don't know what is normal for pregnant women and what is not. They may try to err on the side of what they perceive to be safety, like Marissa's co-workers. However, their delivery as recounted below obviously left a lot to be desired, and Marissa felt infantilized and hurt:

> I had to carry a (maybe) 15-pound package to the warehouse, a distance of 40 to 50 feet. Halfway there I ran into a warehouse employee and asked him to take it the rest of the way since he was heading back there anyway. He started to scold me, telling me that I shouldn't be carrying stuff, just as another co-worker yelled my name and ran up to me to scold me as well. What? Should I just let my muscles atrophy? It's 15 pounds, the weight of a small dog, and I'm not carrying it miles. Also, I'm *full term* and *healthy*. There is no risk. I am not straining myself at all. I

guess moms out there who are pregnant with their second child while their first hasn't yet learned to walk just drag the kids from place to place? The worst is that I was scolded like a child. I joked that I have to build up my arm muscles to carry a baby around but I was really hurt.

And finally we have the co-workers who just can't seem to understand what is an appropriate question and what is not, as Amanda learned:

An acquaintance at work (if you can call someone an acquaintance when you're not actually sure of her name) walked past my desk and asked how far along I am (eight months), and if this is my first child. I said this was my second, and she noticed a photo of my son on my desk. She asked how old he was, and I said two.

"Wow!" she said. "You don't waste any time! Was this planned?"

Why do people feel it's appropriate to ask whether or not this was a planned pregnancy? My husband joked later that I should have told her "Nah, I just REALLY love unprotected sex. I can't get enough!"

Why do all these strangers keep touching me and making comments about my body and pregnancy? It's driving me crazy!

IT'S BIZARRE, ISN'T IT? The moment a woman announces her pregnancy or begins to show, it seems everyone has public access to her belly and an opinion. Pregnancies are public events nowadays. Gone are the times when a woman went into seclusion at 12 weeks and emerged with a squirming baby in her arms.

It does make a certain kind of sense, though. Deep down, in the very smallest corner of our monkey brain, we are all animals with a vested interest in propagating the species. Unfortunately, this often comes out as proprietary or rude. In our opinions, the only things that are appropriate for strangers to say to a pregnant women are "Congratulations" and "You look lovely." Anything else is open to interpretation and is crossing boundaries. Andrea's story below is definitely an example of the latter:

> When I was pregnant, I was waiting on the subway platform and was lectured by a random woman for being a teen mom. A few things: 1. I am twenty-eight years old. 2. None of your business, Lady.
>
> It was intense though. I was very confused! She was telling me that since I had to have that one moment of pleasure, I'll never finish my education and wind up being a welfare queen. She went on to say that I'm bringing my child into an awful life because I am selfish and now she'll be the one supporting me with her tax money, and I better go find the father and marry him since that's the only way to bring up a child.
>
> I literally could not get a word in. The subway station was packed with people who were all staring at us. The lady was *loud*. Finally I shoved my hand in her face and screamed at her that I am twenty-eight years old! I have a college degree! I am married! She just walked away. I still feel really awful about the whole ordeal, since I feel like no woman should have to explain herself to anyone, let alone a random person on the subway. I wish I'd been able to get her to leave me alone without having to assure her that I am doing things "right" according to her. If I were a teenaged pregnant woman, I might have just cried on the spot.

Here is an example from Kathleen showing that some folks just don't seem to have any manners at all:

> I was on the treadmill the other day, and one of the "regulars"— a middle-aged man who wears very tiny running shorts—came up to me and started on this monologue: "I know I've said it before, but you've stayed in great shape! I mean, from here down [motions to his nether regions] and here up [motions to

his chest], you can't even tell you're pregnant! Even your [makes cupping motion to chest, for boobs], you know, haven't gotten bigger! After that baby comes, that weight is going to melt right off! Your husband must be so proud of you! And lucky! And happy! I mean, husbands of pregnant women are very, errr, patient men, when it comes to . . . well, you know. But your husband! [makes growling noise] He's going to be chomping at the bit when you're finally up for it! What a lucky, lucky guy! Well, I hope I haven't been too explicit. Good luck!"

I just had absolutely no response to this. None at all.

Keeping Calm and Cared For

Are there any strategies for me to stay calm, and not let everyone get to me?

ALICE F. FREED, A professor of linguistics at Montclair State University, has noticed that "From analyzing pregnant women's stories, it becomes apparent that others routinely construct for women what their pregnancy is to consist of—often trying to make it a monolithic experience, whether or not this coincides with a woman's own experience."[1] We have observed this over and over again as our clients move through their pregnancies. There is always someone willing to superimpose and project their view of what you should be doing, saying, or feeling right onto you regardless of your reality.

It's a great idea to do some mental and emotional self-care, so you feel strong and confident in both your body and your decisions. Here are a few strategies:

- Spend time with people who know and love you.
- Take time for activities that leave you feeling nourished and happy.

- Vent with girlfriends when you experience a frustrating interaction.
- Keep a journal.
- Cook a great meal and share it with a friend.

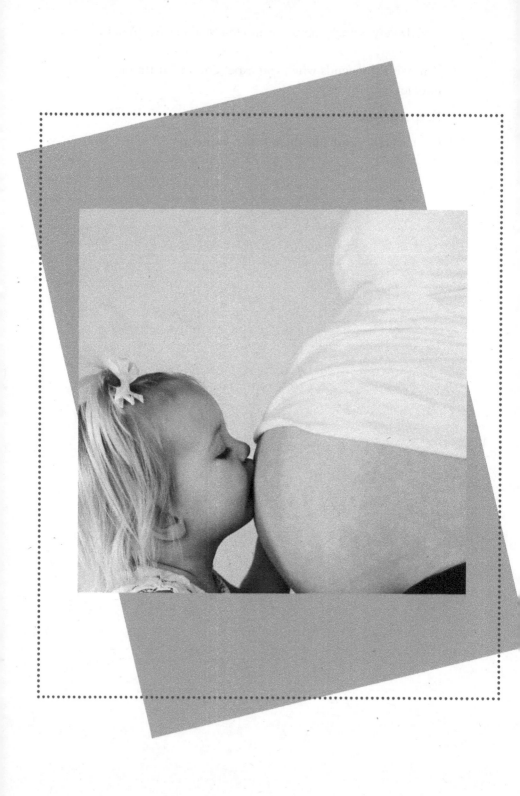

CHAPTER FIVE

She Said, I Said, They Said—Communication

- Anatomy of a discussion
- Informed Consent: Your midwife is talking to you!
- The Birth Plan: Sharing your hopes and plans with your midwife
- Because I said so! Communicating with your family about your choice to homebirth

MAMA SAYS

I respond really well to massage, acupuncture, and sincerity.

—Natasha

Anatomy of a Discussion

THE CHINESE HAVE A saying: "Ninety percent of what we see is behind our eyes." Apply that to daily communication, and we could add that 90 percent of what we hear is behind our ears, and 90 percent of what we type is behind our fingers. We send hundreds, maybe thousands of messages each day, be they verbal, written, or otherwise. We receive at least that many back again. It is inevitable then that we spend a lot of time searching for just the right way to explain something so that it's meaningful to our listener. And if any of these messages are emotionally charged or about a polarizing topic (like, oh, homebirth), we can find ourselves completely blocked from sharing or listening to ideas at all.

We are going to share some general information about communication and then look at one example of how midwives share information—a process called informed consent. We will also look at the example of how parents share information through their birth plans. Finally, we will answer one question that comes up over and over again: How to communicate your choice to homebirth with loved ones.

Can you please define "communication"? What are we talking about here?

WAY BACK WHEN, ARISTOTLE identified three key components to every piece of interpersonal communication: the speaker, the message, and the listener.[1] In Aristotle's model, the most important component is the listener. This makes sense. We could ramble on all day long about our deepest passion. If there is no one to hear us, we are not communicating. Furthermore, if our listener does not grasp what we are trying to say, the communication is so ineffective, it is considered null and void. So, if we intend to communicate, we must have an audience, know our audience, and then check back in with them to confirm that our message is received as intended.

This simplistic model probably worked well for Aristotle and his friends. After all, they were from the same culture, spoke the same language, and conformed to the same basic values. We in twenty-first-century America have it a bit more complicated. Wilbur Schramm, a communications theorist, recognized this and came up with a more relevant model. He agrees with Aristotle regarding the three parts of communication. However, he recognizes that unless the speaker and the listener find common ground, no real communication can ever take place.[2]

In order to share a message that has meaning to all parties involved in a conversation, we rely on finding common vocabulary, experiences, and values. Using all of these elements, along with listening, allows us to move from lecturing others on our beliefs to creating and participating in meaningful conversations.

Anatomy of a Healthy Conversation

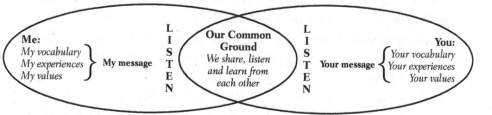

So, what exactly does this have to do with homebirth?

HOMEBIRTH, AND THE MIDWIFERY model of care, are two things that most people have not experienced. Therefore, describing your preferences, perspective, and experiences during this time can be challenging.

Recognizing this can guide the way you talk about homebirth with those around you. Taking the time to build up common ground before you launch into the reasons for your decisions can ease the way for these conversations. Without that common ground, miscommunication occurs. This may lead to anger, hurt feelings, or sadness. It is impossible to have meaningful discussions when one or more of the people involved are in any of those emotional states.

Informed Consent:
Your Midwife Is Talking to You!

I keep hearing the term "informed consent."
What is it?

"INFORMED CONSENT" IS NOT as mysterious as it sounds. Throughout your care, be it prenatally, during the birth itself, or post-partum, you will be asked to make decisions regarding medical tests and procedures. Your health care provider will *inform* you about the tests or procedures. You must grant *consent* before they can be administered. These documents are one form of communication your midwife will use to ensure that you have all of the information you need to make good decisions.

A brief history lesson, if you will: The concept of informed consent is actually quite modern. Prior to the twentieth century, it was generally accepted that doctors knew best, and that they alone were uniquely qualified to decide when and how to treat a patient. This goes all the way back to Hippocrates and the Hippocratic Oath—First Do No Harm.

However, after the horrors of World War II, international outrage demanded a codification of the rights of the individual, particularly when participating in medical research. The result was the Nuremberg Code that was adopted in 1947. It is a ten-point document that details the rights of research subjects and the responsibilities of the medical team. This document was never officially adopted into either German or American law, but it was the first time that patient's rights were explicitly spelled out.

If no laws were adopted, how do I know that my rights
(and my unborn child's rights) are being protected?

IN THE UNITED STATES, four factors govern the practice of informed consent: competency, information, comprehension, and voluntary consent. Be sure that the following principles are upheld when you discuss medical procedures and testing with your provider:

1. COMPETENCY: You must have the ability to understand the conversation, and have the intellectual ability to make the decision.

2. INFORMATION: Your midwife must give you a detailed list of the risks and benefits of each test, treatment, or procedure. In addition to learning what is "normal" for the population at large, you want to learn what the risks and benefits are to you personally given your medical history.

3. COMPREHENSION: You must understand the information given.

4. VOLUNTARY CONSENT: You must not be coerced or under any form of duress. If you are, the informed consent is rendered null and void.

So how does this affect a consumer of homebirth midwifery care?

MIDWIVES TRY TO PREEMPT miscommunication and misunderstandings with written handouts, education, and discussion, that outline the pros and cons of each procedure. In many states, licensed midwives are required to have these documents signed and in your chart. You may ask for a copy to take home, giving you time to reflect and ask questions before signing anything.

Midwives expect homebirthing families to be self-starters when it comes to gathering information, and many families do extensive research on each of the tests. Finding background information is easier than ever before. Gone are the days when we had to sit in libraries poring over medical journals or scrolling through microfiche. Now the latest studies and most up-to-date information are a mouse click away, and most of it is free.

As we mentioned earlier, one of the great aspects of working with a midwife is that most embrace the process of shared learning and decision making. Most midwives we know view it as an ethical obligation to engage in discussions (as opposed to just teaching about the options) with clients when it comes to health care decisions. These discussions are about sharing knowledge and opinions in equal parts from all sources. Parents are more aware than ever of the intricacies of pregnancy and childbirth, and bring to the table a wealth of material and ideas. When our clients come in the door with a notepad and printed-out articles or information, we are thrilled!

The idea is to read the research, talk extensively with your midwife, explore your heart, and then come to a thoughtful, informed decision.

Are there any structured methods we can use when making informed consent decisions?

ALTHOUGH ASKING QUESTIONS OF your midwife should be a given, it can be tricky since sometimes parents do not know the questions to ask, especially early in the relationship. It can be daunting to be presented with what seems to be a momentous choice and have your midwife smile and say, "So, what would you like to do?"

Many childbirth educators use the acronym BRAINS to help give clients a structure to their questioning. It is a method we have seen work well many times. It stands for

BENEFITS: How will this procedure benefit my baby and our family?

RISKS: What are the risks for Baby and Mom?

ALTERNATIVES: What are some other things we might try instead?

INSTINCT/INTUITION: What is your gut telling you?

NOW/NEVER/NOTHING: What if we don't do the procedure right now? What if we never do it? What if we do nothing?

SAFETY/SATISFACTION: Will this procedure increase the safety and satisfaction of the birth for me and my baby?

This first-time father used his BRAINS to decide, with his wife, about testing for group B strep (GBS). This common microbe lives in 10 to 30 percent of women's vaginas, intestines, and rectums, and can be passed to the baby during pregnancy and/or birth. It is the most common cause of neonatal meningitis and sepsis in the United States. According to the American Congress of Obstetricians and Gynecologists, it is fatal to 5 percent of infected newborns, and the vast majority of infected babies do not even become ill.[3] Given this information, Mike and Mara wanted to make a rational, meaningful choice.

> We were really on the fence about group B strep testing. We both come from pretty conventional backgrounds. We had our first baby with an ob-gyn in the hospital, and really weren't used to this autonomy. I don't think anyone even asked us if we wanted to test last time; our doctor just said that this is what happens at this visit, and so we did it.
>
> Mara was negative with our first child and we live a very healthy lifestyle. We just weren't sure it was necessary. Plus, for various reasons, we were paying for this pregnancy and its related fees out of pocket, so we wanted to make sure it was worth it, economically speaking. At the same time, we wanted to do everything we could to protect our baby's health.
>
> We read a bunch of stuff on the Internet, and it gave us a lot of background, but it was still hard to know which recommendations were right for us. Our midwife suggested we walk through the BRAINS template together and see what came up.
>
> > BENEFITS: We thought we would know one way or the other whether Mara had group B strep with this test. But our midwife pointed out that this colonization could come and go, so even if Mara were positive today, she might not be at birth, and vice versa. That was frustrating, because it seemed like we could never know for sure.

RISKS: We couldn't see any risks to the testing procedure. It is a small vaginal swab, like an oversized
Q-tip, which is inserted into the vagina and swiped
over the rectum. It's painless, and Mara could do it
herself at the midwife's office. However, if Mara tested
positive, the standard treatment is IV antibiotics during
labor. That posed some real problems for us. First, Mara
hates needles. Being hooked up to an IV was one of
the things she absolutely hated last time in the hospital
and was one of the reasons we chose homebirth. Also,
we aren't too into antibiotics. We avoid them whenever
we can, because they kill off everything, even the good
bacteria in our systems, and lead to increased antibiotic
resistance. And, as we learned, the test doesn't help us
know if she really will be positive at the time labor hits.
She could be getting an IV and antibiotics for nothing,
and we would never even know. We identified another
risk. If we transferred to the hospital, they might want
to keep our baby longer to observe for signs of infection if we couldn't "prove" Mara was negative by showing them test results. As far as the baby goes, I thought
that if we did do the antibiotics, it would guarantee us
a healthy baby. Turns out, this isn't true. Some babies
get sick even with the treatment. It seems like nothing
is clear about this.

ALTERNATIVES: Aside from deciding whether to test
or not, the alternatives had to do with which treatment
to choose if she were positive. Our midwife told us about
a protocol they use in Europe called a chlorhexidine
wash, a simple douche Mara could use during labor.
It has apparently had very good results in decreasing
the number of early-onset GBS infections in newborns,
and to Mara's delight, there are no needles involved.
She also recommended a very healthy diet, with lots of
immune-boosting foods like garlic, but we tend to do

that anyway. Mara wondered if she could skip the test, but do the douche anyway as if she were positive, for peace of mind. Our midwife agreed to this idea, and so we kept that option on the table.

INSTINCT/INTUITION: We got really focused on the 5 percent of babies who die from this. It felt like a high number to me. I'm a second-time father, and I know how quickly your heart and spirit get very invested in your baby. Within a few seconds of my daughter's birth, I knew I would quite literally die for her. The thought of anything happening to this baby . . . I just couldn't take it. Our midwife explained that if Mara had strep B, there was a 40 percent to 70 percent chance she would pass it on to the baby. Of those infected, 1 percent to 2 percent of babies will show symptoms; and of *those* babies, 5 percent will die. That's a lot less than I had first thought, since I was picturing 5 percent of all babies. But still, I think even one baby is too many.

NOW/NEVER/NOTHING: Our midwife tests for this between 36 and 37 weeks. We could wait if we wanted, but it took a few days to get the results back from the lab, and at that point, Mara could go into labor.

SAFETY/SATISFACTION: We felt that this test would keep our baby safer, even if the results could be potentially uncomfortable for Mara.

In the end, we did test, and Mara was negative. But we still watched our baby very carefully for signs of infection, just because of all we had learned during this process. Well, I think we would watch him carefully anyway. That's what new parents do—we just knew more about what to look for.

—Mike

Each test and procedure has its own ups and downs, risks and benefits. True informed consent does not come easily; wading through the studies and analyzing every possible outcome with your midwife can be exhausting, and there may be no clear-cut answers. Mike's frustrations with the limitations of the GBS test come through loud and clear.

The most important questions parents have to ask themselves are "What am I going to do with this information? Will knowing the outcome of this test change how I am preparing for my unborn baby? Will it give me some clarity or peace that I am missing now?" Then listen to yourself, discuss it at length with your midwife, and trust that you have made the best possible decision in that moment, given all the information you had.

The Birth Plan: Sharing Your Hopes and Plans with Your Midwife

A BIRTH PLAN IS an opportunity to capture your hopes and ideas for your ideal labor and birth and to communicate those to your midwife. We believe there are many benefits of writing a birth plan. This process should inspire you to think about what is important to you and to ask a lot of questions.

Why call it a birth plan when I have no way of actually planning my birth?

GOOD QUESTION! OF COURSE it is difficult to plan the timing, methods, and options that will occur from the first contraction until you are tucked into bed and cuddling with your newborn. The purpose of developing a birth plan is to identify your preferences. Your birth plan serves as a reference guide during labor, allowing you to identify key elements that you would really like to experience. Aim for your dream birth while being flexible. If unexpected events occur, it is much easier to adapt and to not feel let down if you have taken the time to think about what you would want in different scenarios.

If I can't actually plan this birth, and I'm not in charge, who is?

BIRTHING IS A TIME when your body and baby will work together to bring about life. As for who is in charge, your midwife is responsible for your and your baby's physical safety and well-being. She should communicate how she will keep you and your baby safe and healthy well before your labor begins. However, you are ultimately responsible for decisions about your labor and birth.

Even so, your miraculous body will take the wheel. As labor initiates and progresses, hundreds of changes take place within the physiology of your body. The combination of uterine contractions and your baby moving down into your pelvis and putting pressure on your cervix creates a cascade of systemic changes. Your digestive system slows, oxytocin receptors come online, and hormones increase at the right time in the right amounts. You become internally focused and will move in response to your baby's shifting positions. And this is only the tip of the iceberg. (Dr. Sarah J. Buckley's book *Gentle Birth, Gentle Mothering* is an incredible resource for understanding more about these processes.)

It is in the surrender that the process and progress happen. Ina May Gaskin talks about tapping into our "monkey brains." She is referring to the fact that, in order to let the exquisitely formulated cocktail of hormones that drive the birth process do their work, mothers need to be willing to accept that their mind can't control this process. Their skills as planners, managers, and coordinators only get in the way.

So who's in charge? You and your baby are co-captains for this birth. You get to design the plays and pick the key team members. But the birth, like any championship game, will be full of unpredictable dramatic highs and lots of hard work.

How do I know what to put in my birth plan?

YOUR MIDWIFE CAN OFFER you guidance as to the kinds of information she likes in birth plans. Topics you can cover include:

- the names of your birth team and other people who will be present at the birth
    - *Share their relation to you or their role there.*
- information about pets
    - *Share the pet's name, what kind of pet it is, how friendly or finicky, etc.*
- what kind of involvement you want from your midwife
    - *This can range from very minimal to wanting her with you in the same room for as much of the time as possible.*
- what kind of environment you intend to set
    - *Include requests for the birth team to chat in another room, keep the lights low, the house warm, the shades down, or certain music playing, etc.*
- your plans for pain relief
    - *Do you have a birth tub rented? Homeopathic or herbal remedies? Hot and cold packs for comfort?*
- expectations for monitoring you and your baby
    - *Think about how often you want someone to check your baby's heart rate and take your vitals (blood pressure, pulse, temperature). Talk with your midwife about her normal protocols for these issues and make a plan that is comfortable for you both.*
- the birth
    - *Who do you want to catch your baby? Yourself? Your spouse? Your midwife?*

- newborn care

  + *How do you want your baby to be treated after birth? Share your plans for the timing of cutting the cord, if you want skin-to-skin contact with your baby right away, and which medications you plan to give and which you want to avoid.*

- the event of hospital transport

  + *Many women write separate birth preferences that address the hospital staff in case of transport. One thing to keep in mind is that if you started at a homebirth and moved to the hospital, you probably really need to be there. You are there to use the resources and technology they offer but you won't know the reason you need to go until it happens. We have included a list of what to pack for a hospital transfer in the chapter "Labor and Birth at Home."*

Anna's birth plan included a section to bring with them if they transferred care into the hospital.

Dear Hospital Staff,

If you are reading this, we have just arrived from our home where I have been laboring surrounded by my family and trusted midwife. I wouldn't leave there unless I really need extra support. Thank you for providing that support for me!

My husband is with me today, his name is Andrew. So is our great doula, Kim. My goals for this birth are to remain in partnership with my baby as we labor on in the manner that we need to given the circumstances. If I need an epidural, I don't want it to be too heavy. If I need a cesarean section, I would like my husband and doula to come with me into the operating room. Regardless of how I have my baby, I do not want the cord cut until it has stopped pulsing entirely. Also, I would like to do as much skin-to-skin as possible. I am planning on breastfeeding exclusively, so please, no bottles! I am open minded about this birth process and look forward to hearing your ideas for how I can make it great.

Anna

Dena uses her birth plan to discuss boundaries during homebirth:

I would like to minimize internal examinations. Please do not offer to rupture my membranes, and be careful to avoid it if internal examinations become necessary.

If things aren't progressing well, or baby is poorly positioned, I would appreciate suggestions for movements or positions that may help.

She clearly lets her midwife know that she wants as few vaginal exams as possible (which she has likely read increase her risk for infection and can interrupt the labor process) but that she would appreciate suggestions as the midwife sees fit.

Julia wanted to give a brief overview and chose not to list the details; she clearly feels that her midwife knows her and that she does not need to get into specifics:

This is our first child, and we are looking forward to having a natural birth. We have hired a midwife that we trust implicitly and shared hours of conversations with. We have completed childbirth classes and have read as much as possible to prepare ourselves. We have decided to have a doula present to assist us in staying relaxed and comfortable.

The main areas we feel strongly about are the environment during labor and birth, and being fully informed of any procedures you might think would benefit either myself or my baby.

We want a whole lot of quiet. Our home has dimming lights and we expect them to be off or low. We will have candles and music going as we want to. Our doula will help adjust those things. I have rented a birth tub and it will be set up in our room, where I expect to do most of my laboring. You are welcome to use the kitchen, spare room, and TV room to be with your team, chatter, eat, and have a great time. You are welcome to come and go from my room as you need to for monitoring; just come in quietly!

This format is great for sharing plans. In addition to communicating their preferences, it gives a well-rounded sense of the parents. Many parents share their birth plans and ask, "Is that too rude?" The truth is that in our society, we are not great at directly stating our needs. The birth plan/preferences are the time to let your inner diva shine! It is good practice for birth, where all etiquette will go out the window, not to mention how hard it would be to read through if every line is couched in "please" and "thank you." You can show your gratitude by having open, honest communications with your midwife—she will expect you to clearly state your needs in this document.

Ilana talks about her hopes for how she will receive her newborn:

I would like the baby on my chest immediately after birth and for the first two hours. I want the baby to initiate feeding using self-attachment and do not want anyone from the midwifery team to put my breast in her mouth. We will figure it out together—I am excited to get to know my baby in this new way! That said, I am not afraid to ask for help if I need it.

After the placenta is delivered, please place it in a bowl but do not cut the cord until after the first two hours of life.

We have decided not to use antibiotic eye ointment. We will sign a waiver for that. Please discuss your thoughts on vitamin K and our baby's risk of VKDB [vitamin K deficiency bleeding] with us after the second hour of life.

Ilana is protecting the space around her new family. The first two hours of life are precious ones that parents use to inspect and love their baby, bask in the achievement of the birth, and share the experience of new parenting. She is also addressing a very important theme—that mothers and babies will explore each other and figure out breastfeeding (and so much more!) if left to their own devices. She has tapped into the idea that she wants to be the expert on her baby. This statement lets her midwifery team know what *not* to do while also reminding them that she values their support and will ask for it when she needs it.

Makena had her first baby in the hospital. She had some traumatic experiences that she later concluded were due to poor communication. To allay her fears around this happening again, she addressed them in her birth plan. She credits the Web site thegoodbirth.co.uk with the ideas for the questions she included.

> My husband and I will discuss all eventualities as they arise. Please share any concerns with us as they come up so that we are hearing about them long before they become emergencies. We work best with honest and informative advice. Please tell us the truth and offer us information about research and your experience.
>
> It will help us to process the problem if we know the answers to these questions:
>
> 1. What is wrong?
>
> 2. What do you suggest and why?
>
> 3. What would be the possible outcomes with and without this intervention?
>
> 4. How much time do we have to make a decision?
>
> 5. Are there any other courses of action open to us?

Reviewing this plan with her midwife gave Makena the forum to express her fears and to share how she and her husband learn best. Her midwife ran through a sample scenario so that Makena could feel comfortable knowing that they were all on the same page.

Natasha shares her ideal birth scenario with her labor team. She dreams big, and doesn't forget to include having everyone gathered together at her dining room table to enjoy the fabulous meal she has cooked during labor!

> First I want to say "Hello" to all the ladies and my honey and I am so glad we will all be working together on this joyous day! I

am really excited about this baby being born in our home and with respect, dignity, and love. Thanks in advance for making this come true for us!

Please make yourselves at home; when you get here one of us will show you around and show you where everything is. Please eat, drink, read, shower, bathe, do whatever you all need to do and know that our house is your house and we welcome you being here!

The dog is 16 and my first child, he is very sweet and is named Pirogue, and the cat is 18 and sweet but wants attention all the time, so be warned to just move him out of your way.

I am not going to write detailed instructions because who knows what will happen or what I will want but what I can do is tell you what I am like and things that soothe me and my ideas on what would be helpful.

I would love if this occasion would be a festive one with all of us hanging out and not focusing on every contraction unless we need to. So bring your knitting and books to read and I am hoping we can all end up with a loaf of fresh bread and have eaten a delicious meal together in celebration of our hard work. I want to make a roast or stew and if anyone wants to help me chop veggies in the kitchen then feel free. We will have a camera if any of you want to take a few tasteful photos to capture the general atmosphere—that would be wonderful. But we don't need a million of them or for the photo taking to interfere with the birth process.

I want to stay active and enjoy walking outside, maybe visiting our goat in the backyard. I want to have time in the shower (I love water and hot water). I really respond well to massage, acupuncture, and sincerity. I love to have my hair combed. I probably won't talk much or want to hear much conversation when the labor gets strong. Last time I only wanted Steffen around and I liked the quiet. But we will see how it is this time.

Remind me to breathe and to relax/open my mouth and not be tensing up. I am bad about remembering to do these things.

I want to use the tub filled with the hottest water I can have.

Last time it was the only thing, besides breathing and look-ing into Steffen's eyes, that brought me any pain relief. I really like the room darkened and candle-lit if possible. I have a few cds that are background noise/mellow/yoga-ish and we can put these on and see how it goes. If it is nighttime or cold, I would love Steffen to make a fire for me to hang out in front of. I want to sit on a blanket, do yoga, relax, and breathe.

If I start to get bitchy or say I can't do it or it hurts, please remind me firmly that everything is fine. Tell me that I'm doing well and this is what I wanted and that I can do it. If I am being stubborn about it, make me get up and let's try something new for awhile; I will get over it and be happier.

When the baby comes out, I want Steffen to catch her if he wants to and he can pass her to me. When the placenta comes out and it's time to cut the cord, Steffen or our son can do it if they want to.

Please wait until the cord stops pulsing to cut it. We are keep-ing the placenta to make medicine out of it so please rinse it off while wearing gloves and place it in a large ziplock bag. Many thanks!

After the birth, we can all eat something together. I really want to drink something yummy (depends on the time of day, coffee or bubbly or tea) and then go to bed and snuggle up with all my family and enjoy this amazing day. If someone will take a few pictures, I would be grateful as I would like just a few of the new family and of you ladies, as you helped to make this day happen.

Natasha's husband, Steffen, added his own words at the bottom of her birth plan:

During the last birth we did not have any help. We did not know what the best positions were, or how to massage Natasha to reduce her pain. While I will provide the emotional support for Natasha, I would like your guidance finding positions that work for Natasha and showing me what areas to massage and how to massage them. Natasha can get quite opinionated (especially if she is in pain) and does not necessarily listen to me. During that time I need help encouraging her to try different positions. While I respect Natasha's wish to be in the room alone with me, I know that labor can be long and that I do not know everything that will help her. It is therefore fine with me if you are in the room with us or even take over for a while.

I am open to catching the baby and cutting the umbilical cord when the time comes but I know we are playing this all by ear, so just ask me what I want to do in the moment, and I will let you know.

Because I Said So! Communicating with Your Family About Your Choice to Homebirth

My family keeps telling me that homebirth is not safe; how do I talk with them about this issue?

IT IS NEVER EASY when your family is challenging your hard-thought-out decisions. Many couples find themselves rehashing this topic with their family several times over the course of their pregnancy. If you and your partner are in agreement about the plan to homebirth, it helps to strategize and develop some specific talking points. Then it all falls back to basic communication skills. Take a deep breath and share what you know in the best way you can. Speak from a place of honest intent to showcase how you came to this decision and why you are sticking with it. Developing an understanding of another perspective does not mean that you have to change your plans. It just demonstrates your capacity for empathy for others while maintaining your values.

Here is one formula we recommend:

- Say in one or two sentences why this homebirth is important to you.

- Throw in a few safety statistics.

- Remind them that you appreciate their love and concern, and ask them if they have any questions for you. Answer their questions honestly and don't be afraid to say, "We don't know." You can find the answers and get back to them later.

- Summarize your plans in one or two sentences.

Work together with your partner to develop your talking points and role-play. We are including some recent homebirth safety information that you can use for examples, but there is plenty more available. Don't be shy about asking your family to join you at a prenatal visit. As you will read in Kathy's story following, grandparents-to-be are welcome and your midwife will understand their questions and address their concerns. We have seen hesitant grandparents-to-be melt when they observe the quality of care and kindness that a midwife shows to their daughter. This is a place that midwifery care really shines. The long appointments give you plenty of time to show off your midwife's skills, knowledge, and compassion.

Some recent research regarding homebirth has shown the following:

- Out-of-hospital births had similar perinatal outcomes to hospital births and fewer interventions.[4]

- There are similarly low rates of perinatal death in midwife or obstetrician-attended hospital births and planned homebirths attended by midwives.[5]

- Women in the homebirth group were less likely to suffer from postpartum hemorrhage and severe tears.[6]

- Babies of women planning a homebirth were less likely to have low APGAR scores at one minute and the babies were less likely to need drugs for resuscitation.[7]

- Homebirth in a low-risk population does not have increased risks of admission to the NICU or higher perinatal mortality rates.[8] This is important because it brings up the issue that your midwife will assess you throughout pregnancy and screen you for the kind of risks that would bump you into more specialized care.

While these statistics are the most recent at the time of print-ing, a new publication titled *Homebirth: An Annotated Guide to the Literature* provides regular reviews of published literature regard-ing homebirth.[9] You can find it online in several locations, including washingtonmidwives.org.

A few times in life—if you are very, very blessed—you meet people who change you forever. They touch you so deeply by their selflessness and giving that you are never the same. Our midwives were women like this. After what seemed like an im-possible search for a natural birth experience for my daughter-in-law, we came to the door of a beautiful midwife. This was a woman who had made it her life's mission to help women enjoy a normal, natural vaginal birth after a c-section.

My daughter-in-law (whom I will call my daughter for the rest of this piece, because in my heart of hearts she is) had experienced two previous c-sections. She had been erroneously told by her doctor that the c-sections were "required" because her babies were "too large" for her body to birth. We had been informed during her second birth that the hospital, at her insistence, would "allow" her to labor and *if* all went well, she might be "permit-ted" to have a vaginal birth. After a horrible hell-on-earth hospi-tal experience, where my grandson suffered drug-induced fetal distress, my daughter was rushed into her second c-section.

No one tells you about how difficult the recovery period is after major abdominal surgery, let alone while trying to care for and breastfeed a newborn infant. No one tells you about the in-describable pit of postpartum depression that can follow, when these mothers are so fatigued and their hormone balances are so disrupted due to countless drugs, and the interruption of the natural birth process.

After the c-section, the doctors and hospitals collect their big insurance checks and the mothers are sent home to fend for themselves. They are asked if they "have help" at home, but no one checks up on them to make sure they truly do, or if the care is of sufficient quality or duration.

Three years later, when my daughter found out she was pregnant with her third child, I remember feeling what it must have been like for Mary and Joseph on the night Jesus was born. I felt like there was "no room in the inn" for us. No hospital or birth center in our state would accept my daughter-in-law as a patient for a vaginal birth after two c-sections.

When we found our midwife and were introduced to her team, we felt enveloped in a huge hug of hope. Confidence grew each visit, as we asked every question imaginable, and found satisfactory answers. These women treated us like friends—they listened to my daughter and heard the cry of her heart. They lovingly cared for me too, knowing how worried I was for her. Homebirth after c-section can be frightening when you have only listened to the "hospital" side of the story. But as I interviewed (and yes, *grilled*) these women, they earned my trust. I thoroughly researched everything they told us and, surprisingly, found an abundance of truth and studies to back up everything they said. They let us stay as long as we needed to at each appointment, and were patient, kind, and caring.

When it came time for my daughter to give birth, everything was as the midwives said it would be. There were no surprises or disappointments—no "bait and switch" tricks, like had happened in the hospital at her previous birth. The labor was very long, as the midwives had warned us it could be. They monitored the baby's vital signs continually and carefully, and kept reassuring us that the time it took for this baby to be born was "as long as it would take."

No hospital would have "allowed" her to labor for this many hours. But because the midwives had encouraged my daughter to stay fit and healthy throughout her pregnancy, she was therefore able and strong enough to make it through all the difficult hours of labor. My daughter's precious doula stayed with her for every single contraction. They kept her hydrated and well fed throughout her lengthy labor (another thing most hospitals don't "allow"), keeping her strength steady. When we welcomed a healthy and beautiful little boy into the world, with soft music playing, by candlelight (my daughter's birth plan carried out to a "T"), it was as if God Himself entered that room. It was the most intensely holy moment of my life up until that point. Her recovery was amazing, and this little baby was so quiet and peaceful. He didn't suffer the drug withdrawals, colic, and difficulty breast-feeding her previous c-section children had endured.

When my daughter became pregnant with her fourth child two years later, we were so thrilled and thankful to go back to our "safe place" with the midwives. Her pregnancy was healthy and carefully monitored. Again, we felt the same attentive care and concern as we had with the previous birth. They told us that this birth would go faster, and by this time I had learned not to question these gifted birth ladies. The birth was "textbook," as one of the midwives said. Again, here was a second perfect and normal vaginal homebirth, after two previous c-sections. These were large babies and there were no episiotomies required. The doctors and hospitals said it couldn't be done. And here we were, with yet another miracle in our arms (this time a little girl!).

The midwives were the "attendants"—the helping, guiding hands. They guided the baby into the world, and then to the mother's breast. They didn't interfere by weighing, washing, or vaccinating (they did these things many hours later). They left mom and dad with their baby, bonding and falling in love with this new life. They laughed and cried with us, they fed us and kept us warm. I saw them as God's handmaidens—the servants of birth. They let birth and mother and child take center-stage. There was no protocol like in the hospital—no set agenda—no time constraints. Birth called all the shots. They trusted a woman's body to birth her child. They trusted the child to know when to come. It was the closest thing to perfection I have ever witnessed. I will never be the same after experiencing this true miracle of birth afforded to us by these women. They became like dear friends, sisters, daughters, and mothers to me—all aspects of womanhood in one perfect package. These midwives profoundly touched me and my son and daughter-in-law. They touched our deepest hearts. They held our fears in their hands and gently alleviated each and every one of them. I will forever be grateful to them, and I will never forget their kindness. I will never forget their honor and respect of birth. They let themselves be used by God to care for the unborn, the mothers who birth them, and their grandmothers, too!

—Kathy

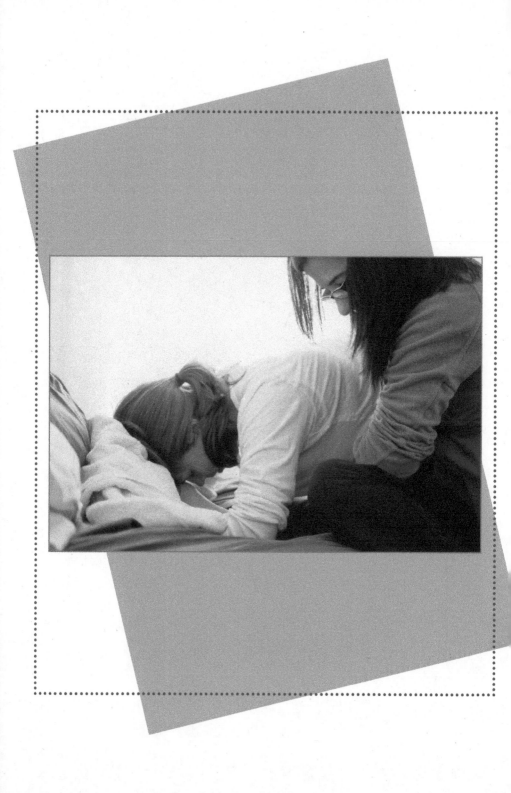

CHAPTER SIX

Your Expanded Pregnancy and Birth Team

- Homebirth and your expanded team
- Childbirth education classes

MAMA SAYS

Our doula, Monica, held my hand, my hair, and our space. She wiped my forehead, my eyes, and my kitchen floor. When it was all over and done, she slipped away like she was never there.

—Lila

Homebirth and Your Expanded Team

CHILDBIRTH EDUCATORS, LACTATION CONSULTANTS, and doulas—oh my! You probably had no idea how many professionals cater to pregnant women until you found yourself in the family way. As you read magazines, browse the Internet, or receive advice from friends and family, you develop an awareness of the vast support and services available to pregnant women today. These services are often heavily marketed by persistent people—some great, some not so great. We know it can be overwhelming and discomfiting—wasn't it just a few minutes ago that you were staring at the little pink strip on the home pregnancy test? How did so many people, who don't even know you, find out about your pregnancy?

Today, expectant mothers have more access to information and support than ever before. No matter what your circumstances are, you don't have to do it alone or feel isolated. When you ask for help, these people and services offer wonderful opportunities to shape your experience. But before you ask your girlfriends who you need to work with and why, do some reading and then sit quietly. Imagine the weeks leading up to your birth—your belly round with baby and your mind and heart full of love and anticipation. What kind of information do you want to know or have access to? What kind of people do you want around you? How do you want your body to feel? How will tapping into these resources support your dreams for this pregnancy and birth? This can guide you when sorting through the variety of care available.

But I'm having a homebirth with a lovely, caring midwife. Do I need to work with anyone else?

YOU HAVE A MIDWIFE. You love her, and she loves you. Isn't that enough? Didn't you decide on the midwifery model of care so you could keep things simple, distill your birth experience down to what really matters? Do you really need all of these extra people?

Well, yes and no. Doulas, lactation consultants, massage practitioners, chiropractors, prenatal yoga instructors, acupuncturists, and other alternative health care providers all offer something unique to birthing women. It's up to you to evaluate each service on its own merits. Does it make sense to you? Can you see the benefit to you and your family? Does it solve a problem you have, anticipate having, or have experienced in the past? Does it make you smile? You get to decide if the care they provide is right for you.

I googled "doula." Now I'm all confused! What's a doula?

A DOULA IS A birthing coach, an extra pair of hands, and sometimes the partner you wish you had. These amazing folks are experts at providing physical and emotional support during labor and the first few weeks of your baby's life. Need your water glass filled? Your doula is on it. Don't think you can push through one more contraction? Your doula can talk you through it. Having back labor? Your doula will have lots of amazing ideas to help ease the pain.

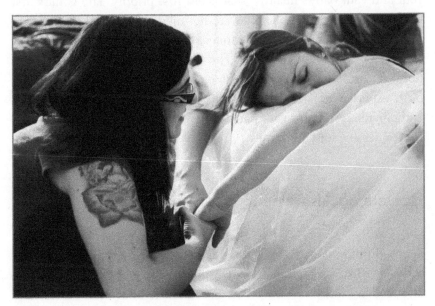

There is nothing like the loving support of a great doula.

In a hospital birth, your doula will be the only professional who is with you through the entire labor, unlike the nurses and doctors who typically leave when their shift is over. A doula can interpret the medical jargon and make sure you are aware of all your options. A great doula will be familiar with each hospital's policies and protocols and can help you work through them.

At a homebirth, your doula will join you in early labor, likely several hours ahead of the midwifery team. She will remind you that what you are doing is normal and healthy, and she will help keep you nourished and strong for the work that lies ahead. In this casual, relaxed setting, your doula can concentrate more on your physical comforts, especially keeping you well fed and hydrated. She can tidy up your house, make a meal for your family, or even take photographs.

So what exactly is the difference between a midwife and a doula, then? Don't midwives do all that?

SURE WE DO. BUT we are also legally and morally responsible for your and your baby's health—that is our first priority. The doula's first priority is your comfort. Doulas are not medical providers. They cannot interpret your baby's heart tones, take your vitals, start an IV, or make decisions about your care. Those are your midwife's responsibilities. We can vouch for the incredible contributions doulas make to the birth experience. The doula's ability to meet your immediate needs and provide respite for your partner or support person creates uninterrupted service for your family.

How are doulas trained?

DOULAS ARE TRAINED IN many different ways. This is not a licensed profession in any state, so basically anybody can call herself a doula. Most professional labor-support people, however, will have attended a workshop, observed a childbirth education series, and attended a certain number of births. The births can be in a hospital or out of hospital, and the medical team and parents evaluate the doula-in-training as she works. If she chooses to be a certified doula, her work is assessed by her certifying agency. Certified doulas must participate in continuing education to maintain their certification. Most doulas participate in online professional groups, where they keep up with the latest research and network with other birth professionals.

If anyone can call themselves a doula, should I worry about certification?

THAT'S A VERY PERSONAL issue, both for the doula and the parents. We know many fabulous, qualified, experienced doulas who have chosen not to certify. Some feel that the agencies' standards are too limiting, and they wish to be free to practice in a less constrained way. Some may not have the financial resources to keep up with the recertification process, which can get quite expensive when you include continuing education workshops, travel to conferences, and other requirements. Research about doulas has shown that it is the presence of a loving woman in the birth space that creates safer, faster, and more satisfying birth experiences. Any loving woman will help you achieve these objectives, regardless of their training and background.

Some doulas and families feel protected by having an organization's endorsement and oversight. A certificate guarantees a certain standard but does not make a great doula.

Regardless of your doula's certification status, make sure she fits into your family and into your heart. Picking a doula based on the number of births she has attended, how long she has been in practice, and if she knows your midwife is a great start. But the most important thing is that you like her. Do you feel comfortable with her seeing you in all your puking, naked birthing, goddess beauty? Does she respect you and your choices in this birth? We recommend interviewing three doulas. One of them will feel like a perfect match.

I want a doula! Where do I start?

HERE IS A LIST of the major doula organizations in the United States. However, don't overlook your local doula groups. Running a quick Internet search of "Doula, [Any City]" will also bring up dozens of options.

> International Birth & Wellness Project (ALACE)
>
> Birth Arts International
>
> Childbirth and Postpartum Professional Association (CAPPA)
>
> Doulas of North America (DONA)

We also recommend taking a look at doulamatch.net, developed by a Seattle doula and childbirth educator. It is a virtual clearinghouse and can provide you with one-stop shopping when searching for doulas to interview. It is designed to help expectant families find doulas who are available during their due dates. It also provides information about each doula's training, certification, and experience levels.

When asked to describe Sharon, my husband says it best: "She was our *guide*." Sharon lovingly helped guide us through cesarean recovery, a miscarriage, surgery for an ectopic pregnancy, and, ultimately, the hard decisions about where and how to pursue a hands-off yet fully supported vaginal birth after cesarean (VBAC).

Over the last three years, Sharon answered all of my tear-filled phone calls and gently yet firmly handed me the shovel when I needed to dig deep. When we were finally expecting our second son, Sharon was an enthusiastic supporter of our strong baby and in my inherent ability to birth him. We initially planned a hospital VBAC, but began to feel unsettled with our decision. Sharon was there every step of the way and, while she never told us what to do or how to do it, we knew that she would go to the mat for us in whatever choice we made. We ultimately decided on what we lovingly refer to as our home GBAC (Garage Birth After Cesarean—my mother-in-law's converted garage) and I have Sharon to thank for believing in me before I believed in myself.

On the day of our son's birth, Sharon was the first person I called to let her know that things were different. She timed my contractions while I relaxed at home in the bathtub and focused on the journey. Once we realized things were hopping, Sharon was instrumental in rallying the troops. She was the first to arrive at the house, and she took care of organizing the labor tub crew to set up and fill the tub. I was in active labor when we arrived and dove straight into Sharon's strong embrace. She was an ace at reading my cues and body language as I was firmly ensconced in "laborland" and unable to speak. Sharon and my husband had a great rapport and had several rounds of priceless banter that still get me laughing. She was equal parts comforting, uplifting, and downright funny!

Our childbearing journey was a rough and tender road and Sharon helped pave the way to a perfect, simple, and powerful GBAC. We are thankful to Sharon from the bottom of our ever-grateful hearts. We did it!

—Janya

What is the difference between a birth doula and a postpartum doula?

SO FAR WE HAVE been talking exclusively of birth doulas. However, there are doulas specifically trained in postpartum family issues. This could be as simple as caring for the baby as the mother catches up on sleep or takes a shower, or as complex as assisting with medically fragile infants. Postpartum doulas can be of great help with twins and establishing breastfeeding. Many of the same professional organizations train and certify both birth and postpartum doulas. In some cities on the east coast, the folks that do the work of postpartum doulas are known as baby nurses.

How about breastfeeding support?

WHILE BIRTH AND POSTPARTUM doulas can provide excellent support during the early days of breastfeeding, there are trained professionals who work exclusively with breastfeeding challenges. Most commonly known as lactation consultants or breastfeeding educators, they provide excellent in-home services for new mothers and babies.

La Leche League International (LLLI) provides comprehensive support that is easy to access. LLLI's mission, according to their Web site (www.llli.org), is "To help mothers worldwide to breastfeed through mother-to-mother support, encouragement, information, and education, and to promote a better understanding of breastfeeding as an important element in the healthy development of the baby and mother." Many a new mother's sanity has been saved by a late-night call to her local LLLI leader. We recommend you attend a meeting during your pregnancy or place a call to your local chapter, just to get a sense of who these women are and what kind of services they provide. The peer-to-peer support from women who have successfully nursed can be invaluable.

Sometimes, however, you need to call in the big guns. An International Board Certified Lactation Consultant (IBCLC) is at the top of the food chain. They have passed a rigorous examination, amassed hundreds of hours of actual experience consulting, and spend all their free time thinking about breastfeeding. Many experienced IBCLCs have more training in breastfeeding than most midwives and doctors. Most IBCLCs are employed by hospitals, but there may be a few independent practitioners. You can find them online at www.ilca.org.

I had a great, fast homebirth, but when my daughter latched on to my breast the first time she breastfed, it was immediately painful. I was a bit perplexed, because I am experienced at nursing. I weaned her two-year-old sister right before getting pregnant. However, on day two when my nipples were cracked and bleeding, I knew I needed help. It was ideal to have a lactation consultant come to my house and help me get the baby to latch on properly. I felt empowered that I knew who to call, and it was nice to have the consultations happen in my home as opposed to a clinical setting. I was propped with my own pillows, on my own couch, with someone I trusted helping me. This gave me extra confidence that I could nurse her without pain and without the stress of getting out to an appointment for help. I saw the consultant twice, and her advice was extremely valuable and useful. Our issues have resolved, and, though nursing my second daughter is still different than my first, I no longer have discomfort. I have a fat, happy baby, and lots of milk!

—Elisabeth

My back is killing me and my hips are all out of whack! Can a massage therapist help?

MANY MASSAGE THERAPISTS SPECIALIZE in working with expectant mothers. Some have advanced certifications, while others come to this work through years of practical experience. If certification is important to you, here are the Web sites of the most commonly seen prenatal endorsements:

www.katejordanseminars.com

www.bodytherapyassociates.com

www.massagedoula.com

www.touchforbirth.com

www.mothermassage.net

There are so many benefits associated with getting regular massage therapy during your pregnancy. Dr. Tiffany Field, of the Touch Research Institute, reports that women who received regular bodywork reported less back and leg pain as well as fewer symptoms of depression.[1] As far as labor goes, women who got regular massage had labors that were an average of three hours shorter, and they reported significantly less pain.[2] Massage increases circulation and it brings a mother's awareness to her changing body. This can be particularly beneficial for those women who may be having trouble integrating these changes and may be experiencing some body image challenges.

Like all massage, prenatal bodywork should not hurt. We are all familiar with that "good pain" that comes from really working out those kinks. But if it is excruciating, please let your therapist know, so she can adjust her technique.

Massage is often covered under health insurance plans, so check with your company. Usually a prescription is required, which your midwife, general practitioner, or chiropractor can write.

What is Mayan Abdominal Massage?

MAYAN ABDOMINAL MASSAGE (MAM) is a relative newcomer to the pregnancy scene, but its star is on the rise. This specialized form of bodywork focuses on the pelvic bowl, and correct alignment of the uterus and other organs. It is based on the traditional work of Mayan midwives and healers from Belize. Brought to this country in the early 1990s by Rosita Arvigo, a naturopathic doctor from Chicago, MAM uses gentle visceral (internal organ) manipulation to ease internal imbalances. This leads to better digestion and reduced PMS symptoms. In pregnancy, MAM provides a greater sense of strength and well-being. It is particularly effective after a cesarean delivery, and while preparing for a VBAC. This work may also reduce scar tissue and break up adhesions, which often form after surgery.

There is a significant emotional aspect to all bodywork, but especially with MAM. If you are not aware of this, it can take you by surprise. The belly is a vulnerable spot for most of us; it is a place we might feel is too big or too small, or think doesn't work right. It is the deepest part of our body, and many of us have learned to guard it with our mind and spirit. Although vulnerable, like our heart, it is relatively exposed—there are no bones or ribs protecting it. Although it can be scary to invite someone into that space, the growth from the experience can be life changing.

You can find certified MAM practitioners at www.arvigotherapy.com.

What about chiropractors?

SOME FORMS OF CHIROPRACTIC work can also be helpful during your pregnancy. Look for a practitioner certified in the Webster Technique. This gentle, noninvasive maneuver shifts the pelvis for optimal alignment. It is one tool we use when a baby is in a breech position to help him turn so that he is head down. According to the July/August 2002 edition of the *Journal of Manipulative and Physiological Therapeutics,* 82 percent of breech babies turned head down after the Webster Technique was applied. You can find more information on the International Chiropractic Pediatric Association's Web site: icpa4kids.com/about/webster_technique.htm.

I love my yoga class. Can I keep going during my pregnancy?

ABSOLUTELY! YOU CAN WORK with your instructor to modify the poses as you get bigger. You can also join a specialized prenatal class, even if you have never tried yoga before.

Yoga can be a valuable addition to any pregnant woman's fitness routine, and it seems especially attractive to homebirthing moms. It may be the candles or the chanting, but we love the emphasis on letting go, following your breath, and trusting your inner guidance. We love the dim lights, and the gentle lengthening of your muscles, and the stress relief, too.

I have been practicing yoga for years; do I really need a prenatal practice?

PRENATAL YOGA CLASSES PROVIDE camaraderie and companionship with other women who are going through the same thing you are. They also effectively help teach you to loosen certain muscle groups in the core as well as your glutes and upper thighs, areas that regular yoga strengthens to unbelievable degrees. The ability to release and loosen these muscles is central to the process of birthing. If they are not released, they act as a hammock (or trampoline) for the baby. We have seen many yoginis suspend their babies on muscles that just will not give way. While eventually it all works out, these labors are the marathons you've heard of in urban legends.

I don't see myself taking a yoga class. Is there anything I can do on my own?

YOU CAN CERTAINLY PURCHASE prenatal yoga DVDs and your midwife can offer you some exercises, but it comes down to spending some time with your pelvis. Tighten your pelvic floor as hard as you can, like a giant Kegel, and then let it go. Do this while holding your breath, and then while breathing deeply. Feel the difference? Now do the same with your glutes and upper thighs. You want to really get to know these muscles, because you will intentionally *not* use them during your labor. You want to be able to turn your lower body into Jell-o at your command. Use imagery, if this appeals to you. Picture your baby sliding down your birth canal with no resistance. Imagine your pelvis opening, spreading, getting wider and wider. Your yoga breathing goes so well with this exercise. Follow your breath down into your body, and picture it going right out your toes, right into the earth. Now you're birthing!

I've heard of using acupuncture in pregnancy. What are its benefits?

CHINESE MEDICINE OPERATES ON the idea that there are lines of energy (meridians) running through our bodies. Our life force travels through the meridians, so we experience our best health when there are no energy blockages in them. Acupuncture is a well-researched, ancient form of medicine with numerous documented benefits. Many of our clients have used acupuncture with great success for a variety of ailments during pregnancy. Some people use it throughout their pregnancy to keep their energy in balance and to address the normal set of muscular and ligament pains. Others use it to address specific issues that come up for them during the pregnancy.

Many mothers have reported a decrease in morning sickness when they receive regular acupuncture treatments. The treatments can be relaxing, and taking a nap while the needles work their five thousand-year-old magic is highly encouraged.

Just be sure to tell your practitioner if you are pregnant. Certain acupuncture treatments can induce labor!

Childbirth Education Classes

Should I take childbirth education classes?

WITHOUT A DOUBT, YES! A good childbirth education class gives you confidence in yourself and your body by explaining the psychological and physiological aspects of labor. A great instructor provides a platform for you to express any fears and concerns you may have, and gives you a safe place to process them before the work of labor begins. Your partner or support person learns positioning techniques, how to help you focus, and what a normal laboring woman looks and sounds like.

Although the classes are primarily educational, nothing beats being in a room full of twenty other pregnant women going through exactly what you're going through. Whether you attend alone, with your partner, or a friend, a comforting camaraderie often develops during the weeks of classes. It's fun to compare notes on swollen ankles, sibling reactions, and the merits of chocolate. One woman got up the courage to tell her class she sometimes dreamed of birthing a puppy. To her surprise, she learned this was normal and even common!

There are a lot of choices in childbirth education. Is there one that covers homebirth?

CHOOSING A CHILDBIRTH EDUCATION class can be a confusing endeavor. Long gone are the days when you just trundled down to the local hospital, pillow in hand (thank goodness!). If possible, we suggest taking a class geared especially for out-of-hospital birth. Check with your midwife, as many educators will leave business cards or brochures with other birth professionals. If this is not available in your area, don't panic. Your teacher will most likely ask where each mother is birthing. If she does not, mention it to her at the break, and she can adapt the information for your situation.

My mom took Lamaze classes in some hippie chick's basement. They did a lot of hee-hee-hooing. Is this what I'm in for?

LAMAZE, WHICH HAS BEEN around since the 1940s, still focuses on breathing techniques, but they offer so much more. These six Healthy Birth Practices form the basis of modern Lamaze classes:

1. Let labor begin on its own.
2. Move, walk around, and change positions during labor.
3. Bring a loved one, friend, or doula for continuous support.
4. Avoid giving birth on your back, and follow your body's urges to push.
5. Avoid interventions when they are not medically necessary.
6. Keep mother and baby together.

We can't find anything not to love here. For more information, see www.lamaze.org.

My older sister and her husband took the Bradley Method; my man is wondering if he wants that much responsibility!

THE BRADLEY METHOD OF Husband-Coached Natural Childbirth prepares couples for a natural childbirth. Some people, including us, are a little turned off by the noninclusive name, but their principles are quite sound. The emphasis is placed on the husband taking a leadership role in the birth experience. This is a great course for couples who really want to learn a lot about pregnancy and birthing. In their comprehensive 12-week-long course, Bradley discusses

1. nutrition

2. physiological changes in pregnancy

3. specific exercises to do in pregnancy

4. the coach's role

5. the first stage of labor

6. the second stage of labor

7. planning your birth

8. variations and complications

9. advanced first stage techniques

10. advanced second stage techniques

11. being a great coach

12. preparing for your new family

This course outline was taken from www.bradleybirth.com. You can find more information there.

How about hypnosis? Can I have a pain-free birth? I like the sound of that!

THERE ARE TWO MAIN hypnotherapy childbirth programs, Hypnobabies and HypnoBirthing. Both offer in-person classes and/or home-study components. Hypnosis is, at its essence, deep relaxation, and there is nothing better than that in labor. These classes remind women that fear can increase pain, and if the fear is removed, the pain lessens or disappears. That said, it is important to remember that pain is a power in our bodies that shows us how to move and what to shift. It can actually be considered a positive and useful sensation of birth. It usually hurts at some point to push a whole human being out of your pelvis. That's okay. We are designed to hurt and then forget it as we are lost in the wonder of the new baby in our arms. We haven't seen anyone who has had a completely pain-free birth using these methods, but we have seen many women with lovely starts to their labor. These programs seem to do best when paired with a standard childbirth education course and when viewed as one of many tools you'll use throughout your labor and birth.

For more information, visit www.hypnobabies.com and www.hypnobirthing.com.

Can you tell me about Birthing from Within?

BIRTHING FROM WITHIN WAS conceived and developed by Pam England, a homebirth midwife from Texas. England believes that an attitude of mindfulness and awareness can be applied to every birthing experience, whether that is a homebirth or a scheduled cesarean. These classes are holistic and intuitive in nature. More information can be found here: www.birthingfromwithin.com.

I found The Pink Kit when I was searching online. Is that a good program?

THE PINK KIT STARTED as a way for mothers to "map" their pelvises with the hopes that a deeper understanding of this great bony structure would generate confidence in the ability to birth. This became a popular activity in childbirth education classes and birth support groups. Over the years, The Pink Kit has evolved into a very practical, down-to-earth childbirth preparation method. It focuses on structural changes you can make in your body to open and create space in your pelvis. We appreciate the biological focus for sure, but it also uses several forms of media to appeal to different mothers' learning styles. There are pages to read, CDs to listen to, and exercises to move to. It is a well-rounded and complete way to prepare for your birth. More information can be found at www.birthingbetter.com.

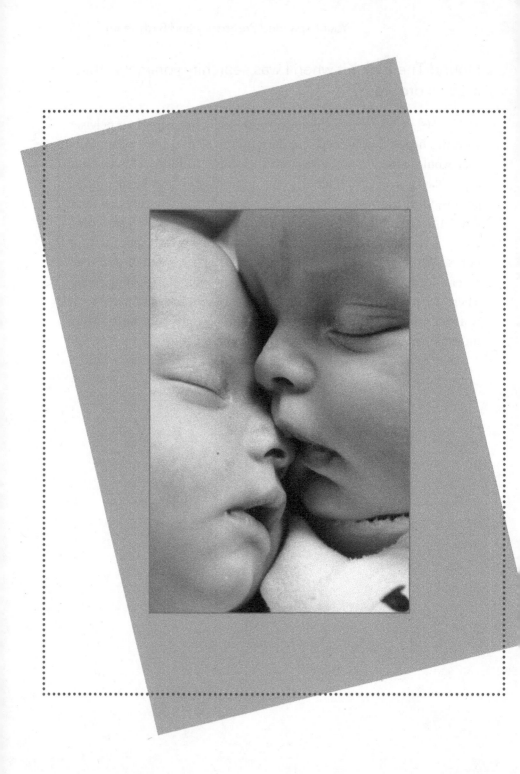

CHAPTER SEVEN

Special Circumstances

- Understanding risk
- Twins and homebirth
- Breech babies and homebirth
- Birth as a sexual abuse survivor
- Teen pregnancies

MAMA SAYS

I was blessed to have a homebirth with twins. I had three midwives and their students attending me and felt that I was in a circle of sisters and mothers. What a sacred way to birth, surrounded by loving and skilled women and my husband. And what a sacred way to be born. Our daughters were welcomed first by us and then by each other. The importance of the relationship they had shared in the womb was preserved during the postpartum time. It seemed as if the midwives could see straight through to the very heart of birth. They kept it protected so that I could do the work of birthing and loving my daughters.

—Victoria

OKAY, BUCKLE YOUR SEAT belts. This could get a bit bumpy. This chapter deals with two special circumstances that may fall outside the comfort zone of many homebirth midwives. They definitely fall outside the comfort zone of many obstetricians. Twin and breech births are hot-button topics in the birth world right now, especially in the homebirth context. There are many providers, of all stripes, who will not accept clients with these particular issues at all, let alone work with them to birth vaginally in their own homes. But this book is not for them; it is for you.

We will also touch briefly on the experience of pregnancy and birth as a sexual abuse survivor, as well as teen pregnancies. While both of these circumstances are routinely seen in hospital birthing, the midwifery model of care offers low-pressure care with acceptance and a gentle guidance that many mothers find to be a good match for their needs. With this kind of support, these moms are more likely to have a healthy, enjoyable pregnancy and to get through labor and delivery without trauma.

Understanding Risk

WE MAKE THOUSANDS OF decisions every day ranging from the mundane to the exotic, and all of them have an element of risk. We are so used to moving through life this way that we hardly even notice. In his book *Beyond Fear: Thinking Sensibly About Security in an Uncertain World*, Bruce Schneier offers five paradigms of risk perception, and how our brains interpret them:[1]

1. Our minds tend to exaggerate rare risks and downplay common ones. Pregnancy is a rare state of being for most modern American mothers. Statistically, most women bear fewer than three children in their lifetime. If you happen to be in a situation where you have twins or a breech baby, your situation is even more unusual. Thus, while nobody worries too much about the risks associ-

ated with showering, for example, the risks of pregnancy loom large.

2. People tend to have trouble estimating risks in unfamiliar situations. For example, when traveling to another city, Americans feel much less safe than they do in their home city, regardless of any real crime statistics. Pregnancy is unfamiliar, and has the added complication of being different every time, especially with twins or breech babies.

3. Personified risks are seen as greater than anonymous risks. What is more personal than your pregnancy? This also explains why your sister's birth experience will influence your feelings and decisions more than any amount of statistics.

4. Our brains like to be in control, and so people will underestimate the risk of something they willingly undertake and overestimate the risk of situations that are out of their control.

5. Most of the time, the media exaggerates the potential risk, especially for newsworthy topics. News stories are aberrations from the norm, or they would not be newsworthy. Nobody pays attention to the millions of healthy babies born every year. But if a mother sees the same study in three sources, say, linking caffeine to miscarriage, you can bet that her barista will be lonely for the next nine months. (By the way, there are mixed study results about caffeine consumption in early pregnancy.)

Once we are aware of how our minds work with risk, common sense tells us that this is how our provider's mind works, too. Each provider has his or her own professional and personal history, just as each mother does. This is true across the board, from the perinatologist at Johns Hopkins, to the unlicensed midwife in the wilds of Alaska, to everyone in between. What is rare or common, familiar or unfamiliar, personal or anonymous, varies with each person. The same is true of the in-control/out-of-control dichotomy, as well as in the news story or Web site we choose to read. All five of Schneier's paradigms work together as each person decides how much credence to give each piece of information.

In America, there are organizations, such as the American Congress of Obstetricians and Gynecologists, the American Medical Association, and the all-pervasive media, that determine how risky certain scenarios or procedures are merely by making a statement. Birth practitioners rely on these sources for guidance. Not only do they accept this information without question (of course there are providers who question what they read, but if and when dissent does occur, it rarely makes the bulletin) but also as a community propagate the beliefs. As an individual, you are sometimes dealing with fact, other times dealing with beliefs, and sometimes dealing with a combination of both. The label "high risk" for your specific pregnancy can be a fact, a belief, or a bit of each.

I have been told I am high risk. How do I decide if it is safe for me to have a homebirth?

YOU GET TO GO through the same process that the providers do. Do your research and evaluate it, being aware of the five paradigms. Read studies and journal articles. Attend support groups. Check out Web sites. Ask your friends for their experiences. Ask any potential providers what their opinions are, and how they came to them. Collect as much information as you can. Notice which factors stand out for you. Do the rare complications make you nervous? Remember, our brain will focus on them. Have you ever had a twin or breech birth before? Unfamiliar situations set off our alarm bells. Do you know someone who has been in your situation? Personal risks seem higher than anonymous risks. Do you feel forced into a certain birthing situation? Remember that we like to be in control, and feel worse about risks when we are not. And make sure you are gathering information from a variety of sources. If we see the same determinant over and over, our brains will perceive it as more risk filled.

Only you can make the decision to homebirth, special circumstances or no. We always recommend that mothers deliver wherever they feel the safest. For some, this may mean their living rooms, while for others, it is the operating room. Whatever you decide, all mothers and babies deserve to be respected in their decision-making process. We trust you.

Twins and Homebirth

I am having twins! Can I birth at home?

YES, ASSUMING YOU CAN find a provider to work with you. Homebirth midwives have to comply with their state's regulations, and each state is different. Some may have restrictions placed on them by their malpractice insurance carriers and/or their professional organizations. Sometimes midwives offer co-care with a physician if they themselves do not deliver twins. This gives the mother the huge advantages of individualized midwifery care during her pregnancy, even if her state requires that she deliver with a physician in the hospital.

How common are twins? It seems like they are becoming more common.

YOU ARE CORRECT. THE rate of twin birth jumped 70 percent between 1980 and 2004, and the rate of triplets and other higher order multiples increased four times between 1980 and 1998.[2] However, this rate is slowing down. The twin rate remained stable during 2005 and 2006, and the level of higher order multiples has declined 21 percent since its high in 1998.[3]

Why the increase?

FERTILITY TREATMENTS ACCOUNT FOR much of the rise, and 44 percent of artificial reproductive technology (ART) births result in twins.[4] In 2006, the American Society for Reproductive Medicine and the Society for Reproductive Technologies changed their guidelines regarding how many embryos can be ethically transferred, resulting in the decline of triplets and so forth.[5]

It is also more common for women over thirty to have multiple babies naturally, and delayed childbearing is becoming more and more common in the United States. Add to this the increased likelihood for obese women to deliver multiples, and you practically have the perfect storm for multiple births.

ART moms are often drawn to homebirth, as it represents a complete departure from the more technological world in which they have been living. It can be a great relief to leave behind the world of daily injections, frequent ultrasounds, and the other trappings that are part and parcel of many babies' conception in the twenty-first century. Birthing at home can be a way of reclaiming that most natural of processes, and giving a human connection to what had previously been a sterile and stressful process.

Can you tell me about the different types of twins?

YES, IT'S IMPORTANT TO know what type of twins you have, because it can impact your care. There are two different types of twins, monozygotic and dizygotic. Monozygotic twins, also called identical twins, are genetically identical and occur when a fertilized egg splits in half. (There are some very rare cases in the literature regarding monozygotic twins who are not genetically identical, but that is beyond the scope of this book.) Identical twins can only be the same sex. It is a common misconception that all identical twins share the same placenta and amniotic sac. Some do, and some don't. Dizygotic twins, also called fraternal twins, are two different eggs, fertilized by two different sperm. These twins are essentially siblings who share a womb. Fraternal twins may be two girls, two boys, or one of each sex.

Apartment Living

Traci B. Fox, an instructor of ultrasonography at Thomas Jefferson University, has a great mnemonic device for keeping the different types of twins straight. She calls it The Apartment Analogy.[6] Twins who have their own amniotic sacs and their own placentas are called dichorionic-diamniotic (Di-Di). They have two completely separate apartments, with their own bedrooms and kitchens. These can be either fraternal or identical twins. Babies who have different amniotic sacs but the same placenta are known as monochorionic-diamniotic (Mo-Di), and can only be identical. These babies live in the same apartment, with two bedrooms and a shared kitchen. Monochorionic-monoamniotic (Mo-Mo) babies share both the sac and the placenta, and again, can only be identical. They are living in an efficiency apartment, with one bedroom and one kitchen.

It is worth noting that sometimes Di-Di twins' placentas can fuse together during pregnancy. These twins are still considered Di-Di. It is also worth noting that these twins usually have the least problems during delivery, and are often the only type that an out-of-hospital provider will consider delivering.

I thought twins and breech are high-risk pregnancies?

"RISK" IS A LOADED word. Sometimes it feels like our entire lives, not to mention our pregnancies, are governed by actuarial tables, statistics, and other people's malpractice insurance policies. If only it were that simple! Real, true risk is very difficult to quantify, and can mean different things to different people. We're sure you have encountered folks who think birthing at home is "too risky" under any circumstance. When pressed, most people cannot really articulate why they feel that way, usually murmuring something about emergencies and "What if something happened?"

What are the main risks in a twin pregnancy?

THE BIGGEST RISK WE see is women becoming disconnected from their bodies and their babies. It is so easy to have that innate connection, that very real psychological and physical bond between mother and children, be reduced to a series of visits, tests, and what-ifs. Many mothers pregnant with twins spend their entire pregnancies preparing for the inevitable problems that may occur during their children's delivery. We are not suggesting that you ignore the risks of delivering twins. However, we also want you to enjoy the miracle of your pregnancy and the babies growing in your body. A few minutes a day spent in quiet meditation or gratitude can go a long way.

Twins have a much higher rate of prematurity (being delivered before 37 weeks). In fact, 60 percent of twins are born prematurely, which may be why so few are born at home.[7] These children often have respiratory, temperature regulation, and other health issues. This also explains the likelihood of low birth weights among multiples, which increases their risk of these same health problems.

Ten percent of identical twins who share a placenta will develop twin-to-twin transfusion syndrome (TTTS).[8] In this rare condition, blood flows from one twin to another, which can cause problems for both. The donor twin is often born anemic and pale, and may need a blood transfusion. The recipient twin may actually have too much blood and also need medical care. TTTS is usually diagnosed before birth, using ultrasound, and most cases are treatable. This condition is outside the scope of a homebirth midwife, although, as mentioned, she may be able to provide parallel prenatal care.

Multiples can strain their mother's body, putting her at greater risk for preeclampsia and gestational diabetes. It is a good idea for you and your provider to come up with a care plan to minimize these risks as much as possible.

What direction should my twins be in? Will this matter if I want to birth at home?

THIS DEPENDS ON YOUR provider. Twins are designated as Baby A (who is closest to your cervix) and Baby B (who is closest to your lungs). It is optimal if both babies are head down. However, many midwives (and doctors who deliver twins vaginally) will consider attending a birth in which Baby B is breech. It may be more difficult to find a provider who feels comfortable if Baby A is breech. The first baby will pave the way for the second, making a twin breech birth easier than a single breech birth.

What does a twin homebirth look like?

IT'S A PARTY! THERE will be at least two midwives and probably three. There will also be an assistant for each midwife. Each baby and the mother deserves her own care provider, and every attendant will be trained in neonatal resuscitation. The same equipment will be present as at the birth of one baby, just twice the amount. You will see two resuscitation stations, consisting of oxygen tanks and masks, a stethoscope, a thermometer, and a heating pad to keep the baby warm. Twins are more likely to need a little help with their breathing, especially the second baby, so this equipment will be close at hand.

The first twin is born in the usual fashion, and if he doesn't need any extra help, can be given to the mother to hold. The cord is cut, and everyone oohs and ahhs while they wait for contractions to start again. There is a chance that Baby B might turn transverse (sideways), so the midwife may apply gentle pressure on each side of your belly to keep her head down. Baby B will be closely monitored by Doppler until she makes her grand entrance. When she is born, there is typically a pause of several minutes before the placenta(s) birth. If either twin needs resuscitation, she can be worked on while the mother is holding her, or if necessary, brought to the resuscitation station and assisted.

After the birth, the mother will be watched carefully for too much blood loss, especially after the placentas are born. There will be extra heartbeat checks for the babies and extra blood pressure checks for the mom. All of the other postpartum procedures remain the same as for any homebirth.

Breech Babies and Homebirth

My baby is breech, what does that mean for birth?

A BREECH BIRTH OCCURS when Baby decides to nestle up under your heart, rather than planting his head down into your pelvic bowl. A wise midwife we know commented that "breech is the second most popular way babies are born." Many babies are breech at some point during their gestation. Only 4 percent are still upside down at term.[9]

Are there different types of breech?

THERE ARE THREE MAIN types of breech positions:

1. FRANK BREECH: The baby's bottom is headed toward the cervix, her legs are straight, and the feet are up by her head. Think of a diver in a pike position. This is the most common type.

2. COMPLETE BREECH: The baby's bottom is also down by the cervix, but this time her legs are crossed. This is the second-most-common type.

3. FOOTLING OR KNEELING BREECH, ALSO KNOWN AS INCOMPLETE BREECH: This time the baby is leading with her foot, or her knees. This is the rarest of the bunch.

I have a breech baby right now, and I am not full term yet. What can I do to encourage my baby to flip head down?

IF YOU WANT TO gently encourage your baby to flip, try lying upside down on a slanted surface such as an ironing board that's propped against a really stable piece of furniture. Be sure to have a spotter. Pregnant women have low centers of gravity. You can also play music nearby your pubic bone, or shine a flashlight down there. Bonus points if you can do all three at the same time! Some mamas have had success with doing handstands in a pool. (At the very least, it feels great to just float, belly down, for a while.) Homeopathic *Pulsatilla* is another option we have seen work. The Spinning Babies Web site (www.spin ningbabies.com) is chock full of different positions you can try to turn your baby. We also recommend talking to your baby and visualization.

At the same time, consider getting your pelvis aligned through chiropractic care. Look for a chiropractor certified in the Webster Technique. It is thought that a misaligned sacrum can pull on the uterine ligaments and cause the uterus to become twisted or torqued. This can force the baby into a position that is not optimal for birth.

Babies seem to love acupuncture, and we have seen some impressive baby-flipping happen after a session. Several studies have shown good results, although the control groups tend to be small. Moxibustion, burning dried mugwort over a certain part of the body, is often a part of the breech protocol.

The most invasive of the breech turning techniques is the external cephalic version (ECV). This involves a care provider, usually an OB, manually turning the baby from the outside. Most times this is done with ultrasound guidance, and some providers even recommend an epidural, since the procedure can be uncomfortable. The success rate of ECV ranges from 48 to 77 percent, with an average of 63.3 percent success.[10] Some doctors are better at it than others—and some babies are more cooperative than others, too!

As with any intervention, there are some risks involved in an ECV: The baby's heart rate can drop, due to cord entanglement or stress; and there is a slight chance that the amniotic sac will break during the procedure. Additionally, the placenta can come away from the wall of the uterus, which is called a placental abruption. On rare occasions, the doctor may recommend an immediate c-section if the baby is not tolerating the procedure well and the heart rate does not return to normal after the ECV is stopped, or if there is maternal bleeding. For these reasons, you and your baby will be closely monitored during the ECV.

I've tried everything, and my baby just won't flip!

THIS CAN BE INCREDIBLY frustrating, especially if you are not comfortable with vaginal breech birth, or this option is not available in your area. Sometimes babies really do know best. There could be a very good reason why your baby won't turn—we may find out the reason during your delivery or we may never know. We strongly believe that babies and their preferences should be respected. They may have an innate knowledge that we do not. There are certainly stories out there of tenuous cord attachments and the like, which could have spelled disaster if a baby's position had been forced to change. If your baby won't flip, perhaps she is not meant to.

This can be so hard to accept and can trigger intense feelings of loss and grief, especially if it means the loss of your homebirth or of your vaginal birth. This is normal and natural. Take the time to really feel these emotions, and share them with your baby. Work through them together, with the help of a professional if needed.

I'd like to deliver my breech baby vaginally, preferably at home. Is this safe?

AH, BY NOW YOU know what we are going to say, right? Only you can make that choice. If you are considering this, we recommend that you connect with a midwife who is experienced in this type of delivery. Some feel comfortable delivering any type of breech. Some midwives, however, only feel comfortable with a frank breech, or with a mother who has already borne a child. Even in the hospital, breech birth is no longer automatically a c-section. However, many new providers, both doctors and midwives, have not been adequately trained in the intricacies of breech birth. Many midwives' malpractice policies do not insure breech deliveries, so of course, be sure you understand all of the ramifications of your choice.

Recently, the Society of Obstetricians and Gynecologists of Canada conducted an extensive literature review of the major breech studies. In March of 2009, they revised their guidelines for breech birth, saying that they no longer support automatic c-sections for breech babies.[11] Yet this landmark revision acknowledges that there is a lack of trained providers for breech birth. There has been a recent upswing in breech birth trainings offered for birth professionals.

What are the risks of a breech vaginal birth?

THE TWO MAIN RISKS of a breech delivery are:

1. CORD PROLAPSE: This occurs when the cord comes through the cervix ahead of the baby. It is much more common with breech deliveries. Footling and kneeling breeches are particularly prone to this, because the presenting part is not big enough to completely cover the cervix. A cord prolapse is less likely with a frank or a complete breech. Because the baby's buttocks fill the cervix, there is no space for the cord to drop through. If the cord comes through the cervix first, it can be com-

pressed, which limits the blood and oxygen supply to the baby. Insufficient oxygen can lead to brain damage or even death.

2. HEAD ENTRAPMENT: The biggest part of a baby is his head. The head will usually come through fine if it is well positioned. Sometimes for reasons we cannot control, it is not and the head can become stuck. There is also a chance that the body will fit through a cervix before it is completely dilated. In these cases the head may not follow easily through the small cervix. Regardless of the reason, a trained provider will have methods to try to release it. Either way, head entrapment can cause fetal distress and, in rare cases, death.

We knew I was having a frank breech baby. We tried all the traditional things to turn her: acupuncture, handstands in the pool, shining a light at my lower body. However, my little girl remained happily upside down. I even went for an external cephalic version, where an OB tried to turn her manually from the outside. She would shift a little bit, but then immediately return to her usual position. I really think that she was meant to come into the world bottom first. I felt really confident that I could deliver her that way, so I started my late-third-trimester search for someone who would help me.

My massage therapist gave the name of a homebirth midwife who had delivered many breech babies. I visited with her, and liked her immediately. She was calm and knowledgeable, and really believed I could do this.

I went into labor on a cold winter's day, around six in the morning. I was grateful that I had had a good night's sleep. I felt energized and excited. The contractions started about seven minutes apart, and they were completely bearable. I was able to get through them by walking and swaying. Soon, they got closer together, and I was starting to lose it a bit. My husband held me and rocked me, and told me I was beautiful. You know, that really works!

When the contractions were five minutes apart, we called the midwife. She said she would leave right away. I was already starting to feel some pressure in my back and bottom, like I had to have a big bowel movement. I went to the toilet, but nothing really happened. While I was sitting there, however, I heard a big splash of fluid come out and felt a "pop!" My water had broken! I was also having a good amount of bloody show, and a lot of mucous. The birthing process so far was proving to be very moist.

The midwife arrived and checked me, and I was almost complete! I couldn't believe it. When she took her hand out of me, there was meconium on her glove. I started to freak out a bit because they had told us in birth class that this could be a sign of a stressed baby. The midwife told me that all breech babies had some of it, as their bodies were being squished on the way down, and there was no place for it to go but out their rear-end. That made sense. Slightly gross, but I understand why.

Soon I started to push. My midwife had me lean back on the bed, with my bottom almost hanging off the edge. She let my baby's butt come all the way out before she gently supported it. I could feel the whole thing! I could feel my baby twisting inside me, working her way out. I felt one leg pop out, and then the other. The midwife gently waited, and soon I felt the arms come through. It seemed to take forever to get her head out, but we had time. Nobody was rushing anything. Finally, she just slipped out. She cried almost immediately, and I held her right away. It could not have been more perfect. I can't imagine giving birth any other way.

—Marilyn

Birth as a Sexual Abuse Survivor

APPROXIMATELY ONE IN THREE women in this country has been sexually abused.[12] Many of these women will seek the comfort and safety of homebirth. In midwifery care, control and autonomy are considered the property of the mother, which can be extremely healing for survivors of sexual abuse. Most midwives are uniquely qualified to offer emotional and physical support for mothers as abuse-related issues arise throughout the pregnancy and birth.

I am an abuse survivor, and really don't like to talk about it. Do I have to share this information with my midwife?

YOU CERTAINLY DO NOT have to do anything that makes you uncomfortable. However, if you feel up to it, sharing your history with your midwife can be helpful for both of you. Chances are she has worked with survivors before. She will listen to your story and likely share some experiences and ideas that have helped other mothers through this time. There is also a lot to be said for just sharing your story—it can be healing to know that you are not alone. Everything that you say will be held in the strictest confidence by your midwife. She is ethically bound to protect the information you share with her.

Many midwives have questions about sexual history and/or past abuse on their intake forms. This often provides mothers with an opening to share their experiences. However, some mothers prefer to wait until they get to know and trust their midwife to disclose their abuse stories. It is fine to take some time to develop this relationship. Trust may come from the moment you realize you want to hire her or it may come gradually. There is no right or wrong answer. You can disclose your history when and if you are ready to share it.

This pregnancy and upcoming birth are bringing up a lot for me. How do midwives approach survivors who are still working through issues?

MIDWIVES WILL MEET YOU where you are in your process of healing. We do not expect you to act like a happy pregnant mother when you are feeling torn up, confused, or angry on the inside. There is room in midwifery care for the expression of who you are in the moment. There is room for you to set parameters and make decisions if they will help you feel safe. There is room for you to question, explore, grieve, or look forward. This idea is fundamental to midwifery care.

Many survivors choose homebirth because it offers them so much control. During pregnancy and birth, there are hundreds of details and decisions that come up. It is up to you how to proceed with each one. Your midwife will help you create and build the scaffolding you need to support yourself through this time.

This book talks a lot about surrender and release, two things I am not very good at. Will I be able to birth?

SEXUAL ABUSE IS ALL about power and control. It is not about sex, intimacy, or any of the other lies that victims have been told by their perpetrators.[13] Survivors have learned that to lose control is to be in danger, and many have structured their lives to avoid this. This naturally extends into pregnancy and birth.

The concept of relinquishing control and giving in to surrender and release can feel daunting and overwhelming—even terrifying at times. With homebirth, letting yourself surrender or release does not nullify the fact that you have control of many aspects of your birth. You have picked your team and your environment. You are releasing yourself to birth within the safe confines of many options that you do control.

Also, surrendering to the birth process is really about establishing a new connection with your body, one where you see your body as a beautiful extension of your spirit. We understand that trust in your body is difficult. But you are not trusting someone or something "out there." You are developing a trust and respect for your body and the fact that it can create and bring forth life without a whole lot of input from you. Your body will do something miraculous for you during birth—it will bring you your child and may provide emotional healing in the process. The concepts that people associate with the words "surrender" and "release" can be quite different from person to person. Sit with them for a while and see if you can develop a meaning that makes sense and is achievable for *you*. Talk with your midwife about this. Maybe together you can reframe these scary concepts.

> I am happy to say that when I did give birth—although it was not easy—it was not violating. And although I felt forces much bigger than me at work, I never felt out of control. In contrast to what I feared, the moment of pushing and helping my baby navigate my pelvis was the most powerful moment of the whole experience. As my baby pressed into the walls of my being, opening impossibly wider with every push, the old story seemed to be forced right out with him. There was no room for the story of a small, voiceless victim. A new story was being written, cell by glorious cell. This part of my body was a place of power, of divine strength. This was a place where miracles happened. This was a home, the beginning of another person's life. This small, perfect boy was remapping the way for me, showing me what femininity was all about. He was teaching me about trust. He was showing me that I could be violated, could give way, could tear in two—all in a glorious celebration of life.
>
> —Katie

Is there anything else I should be doing for this pregnancy?

WHILE THERE MAY BE struggle and hardship as you move forward, pregnancy and birth also bring the potential for growth and healing in your life. Be gentle with yourself; pregnancy is naturally a time when things feel confusing and overwhelming. Continue to surround yourself with people you trust and love. Take your time making decisions. Actively create a space in your home where you will feel safe to do the work of birthing.

The Midwife Says: When we work with survivors, two things leap out at us: the health and beauty of her pregnant body, and the wisdom behind the choices she makes to ensure that she feels safe and protected. We feel called to sit with this woman—to be by her side and love her whole self—the fear, the expectation, the need, the joy, the achievement. They are hers to own, and ours only to witness and appreciate.

I would like to work on myself so I can heal from the abuse before the baby is born. What do you recommend?

THERE ARE SEVERAL OPTIONS for you to explore. You can certainly talk openly with your midwife about your abuse and the areas of your life you would like to heal. Your midwife will have local referrals for therapists or groups that you can contact.

There are two wonderful books on the market targeted for mothers who are sexual abuse survivors. The first is *When Survivors Give Birth: Understanding and Healing the Effects of Early Sexual Abuse on Childbearing Women* by Penny Simkin and Phyllis Klaus. This book discusses the impact of sexual abuse on children, adults, and on all aspects of childbearing. It also teaches skills in communication and self-help. *When Survivors Give Birth* is designed for women and the professionals who work with them, so you will get a glimpse at different healing modalities as well.

The second book is *Survivor Moms: Women's Stories of Birthing,*

Mothering and Healing after Sexual Abuse by Mickey Sperlich, MA, CPM, and Julia Seng, PhD, CNM. This book is full of stories from women just like you. It is insightful to see how other women survivors approached childbirth and what worked for them.

> Labor: That's when I became not only a mother but a grown-up. I really tried hard to take control of it, but I was always aware that I really couldn't. The similarities to my rape just freaked me out. I didn't get to pick when it happened, I didn't get to pick how it would feel. I didn't get to pick anything, just like the night I was raped. I tried, of course. I had a big birth plan, full of the tiniest of details. I would write it and rewrite it, every time I thought of a different labor scenario. In the end, my midwife and I decided I should focus on the things I could control, and I put all my energy into those.
>
> Instead of having major freak-outs about how I would handle my pain if and when I felt it, I settled down. I focused on concrete details. For instance, I knew I wanted a calm, soothing atmosphere. What did that look like? What music did I want to hear? Who was going to be present? These were the little details that I could control, but by focusing on the small stuff, I was able to release the bigger stuff.
>
> This strategy worked really well, and I was able to relax when labor hit. My husband was absolutely amazing at supporting me, and everything turned out great. I've since used this "small stuff obsession" in other areas of my life, and it has worked well with them too.
>
> —Marie

Teen Pregnancies

WHILE ON THE SURFACE this might seem an odd book to discuss teen pregnancies, we have found that teenagers can be highly plugged into birthing outside of the normal institutional methods. We have also seen many examples of how teenagers process their decisions regarding how they want to birth their babies. If you are a teenager reading this, welcome! We are so happy you are here investigating your options.

I am seventeen years old and pregnant. Why might I consider midwifery care?

MIDWIFERY CARE OFFERS TEEN moms extra layers of social support, honest communication, and the deep-seated belief that they will exceed all expectations. Midwives work to empower all mothers through listening, education, and support. Teen moms are no exception to this rule.

Are teenagers too high risk for midwifery care?

A TEEN SHOULD NOT be risked out of midwifery care for age alone. Other risk factors may come into play. If you are curious about whether you are a good candidate for midwifery care and a homebirth, set up an appointment to meet with a midwife. She will consider your medical history and risk factors in the same way she would for any mother. Many midwives are thrilled to work with teen moms. You tend to be really interesting people!

Can my boyfriend be involved in the birth?

OF COURSE! YOU CAN bring him to prenatal appointments and the midwife can show him how to feel the baby in your belly, and he will hear the baby's heartbeat as well as take part in your goals for the pregnancy and birth.

We have seen a few examples of teenage fathers at birth. One of them played video games the whole time until Mom was ready to push. It was his way of coping with the stress. When she started pushing, he was right there at her side encouraging her and saying some very kind things.

Another dad came to all of the appointments and played a huge supportive role during labor and birth. The trick is to find out what role suits your partner best. If it fits with what you want for your birth, great. If not, and you need help finding the right role for him, talk it over with your midwife. Older dads need help figuring this stuff out all of the time. It is normal for men to grapple with finding their place in this very female event.

Nikki struggled to find a provider who was a good fit for her, but her persistence and willingness to communicate with her family paid off:

My pregnancy was a complete and giant surprise. I met with my school counselor and she helped me plan a way to talk to my parents. She even offered to be with me but that didn't seem like the right thing to do. I had a lot going on in my own head— for some reason I was mostly worried about how a baby would fit through my vagina! That fear was worse than the fear of my parents, which somehow helped me get the courage up to tell them. I did tell them and after a couple of weeks of hard times they calmed down and told me that they wanted to be there for me.

My mom made an appointment with the doctor. We went in and she spoke at me like I was an idiot. I felt really hurt and angry. I did a stupid thing, I know, but I'm not stupid in general! I thought, "Great, now I have nine months of this to deal with." When we left, my mom asked me how I liked her. I said, "Fine," because I thought she would get mad at me if I argued and I was, for the moment, on my best behavior. My mom challenged me and asked me to think about the kind of person I wanted to work with. I started to list things that were important to me:

- not a lecturer
- someone who understands that I am capable of making decisions

- someone who is nice

- someone who wants to hear my side

- someone who does not judge me

My mom asked if we could spend some time together when we got home.

We looked online and read a few articles about different kinds of doctors and we also saw some information about midwives. I really liked how they seem to talk to moms as if the mom was in charge. I also liked the messages about keeping it all kind of low-key. I didn't want a lot of strangers around me and was intimidated by having to go to a hospital to "prove" I could do it.

We made an appointment with two midwives to meet them. I liked them both but one of them just seemed like an older sister who knew a lot about birth. We decided to hire her. I felt really great after each appointment. She expected me to be smart about my baby and how I took care of myself. She gave me reading and classes to go to. I didn't want to admit it at the time but everything she told me to do really mattered. I read about all kinds of options every time she offered me a test. She gave me some Web sites to read and I learned about homebirth and hospital births. The entire pregnancy she reminded me that all of my options were open and that she would support whatever choices I made. I could feel that she cared about me. She was amazing at talking with my parents, too. Sometimes we would fight and she would help me see their point of view but she always seemed like she was on *my* side. It felt really great to have someone like that in my life.

I did have a natural birth at home, and it hurt but it worked! I am really glad I did it. My boyfriend was there and for the most part he did okay but I also felt like he kept bugging me and I was thinking a lot about what he was thinking instead of what I was doing. At one point he asked me if I wanted to go to the hospital to get some pain medication and I remember staring at him and yelling, "Dude. I'm seven centimeters; I'll be done soon, shut up!!" It felt kind of good to yell. It was superhard and I am really glad I did it. Now when other girls come to me to talk about what my experience was like, I really try to tell them not to be a lemming and just do what everyone else is. I will always be happy that I found a midwife who treated me like mine did.

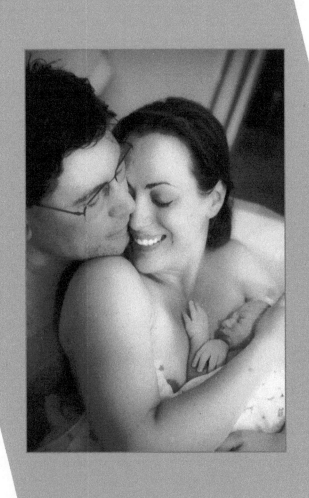

CHAPTER EIGHT

Homebirth After Cesarean

- Why HBAC?
- Is HBAC safe?
- Finding an HBAC midwife
- Finding peer support for HBAC

MAMA SAYS

The only way to rid your mind of fear is to saturate it with truth.

—Michelle

Why HBAC?

WE CONSIDER THIS CHAPTER the living room of our book, as it reflects the heart of our birth work over the past eleven years. So have a cup of tea, put up your feet, and breathe easy. You are welcome here. A Homebirth After Cesarean (HBAC) can provide an empowering and healing experience for mothers and we are thrilled that you are investigating your options.

Many HBAC moms wonder if they are "too risky" for homebirth. Every birthing woman has her own set of risk factors to consider, and HBACs are no exception. We have found that a mother who is a good candidate to consider homebirth is usually a good candidate to consider an HBAC. And just like any other woman considering a homebirth, we hope that you will gather information from a variety of sources and put all of it together to make the decisions that are best for where and how you want to birth.

We believe strongly in the right to HBAC and the safety of these births. That is because we have seen how HBAC mothers prepare

VBAC: A Verb and a Noun

A note about the vocabulary: the terms VBAC (vaginal birth after cesarean) and HBAC are commonly used as both nouns and as verbs in the publications and resources you will encounter. Ours is no exception. Additionally, while we honor the choice to VBAC in the setting you desire, and have attended many fabulous VBACs in the hospital, we will use the term HBAC here as this is, after all, a book about homebirth!

If you are still investigating VBAC versus elective repeat cesareans, please see Appendix D for resources.

themselves prenatally. They work tirelessly to eliminate as many risk factors as they can so that they will be healthy and strong for the work of labor. They wander into the corners of their psyche to prepare themselves emotionally. They ask for honesty and insight from people they trust. And they use many resources to make good decisions. They know that the effort preparing for and the hard work during the actual birth experience are crucial.

My first baby made me a mother. She was a c-section. I loved her, I was present with her. I got busy mothering her and did not consider the way she was born until I was pregnant with my second baby. The thought that I wanted something different sent me on the journey of a lifetime.

I began to want a vaginal birth. I educated myself and found a homebirth midwife who would support me. My husband was a partner in education. I read birth stories and book after book about labor. I watched videos and read the research behind every issue that came up. I stopped eating dairy and sugar (except some occasional ice cream) and walked every day. I was a lean, mean, birthing machine!

I approached the birth like this: I was going to do every single thing that I could in the best way that I could. When I look back at my first birth, I think a lot of why it ended in a cesarean was just plain ignorance on my part. I just didn't know what I could do to give myself the best shot. For the second birth, I felt strongly that if I learned and did everything I could, I would be okay with another c-section.

My second birth pulled me places emotionally and physically that I did not even know existed. It was a real a** whupping! After every contraction (and I do mean *every* one over the course of several hours), I would look at my midwife and ask, "Will this work?" or "Do I need another cesarean?" or "Can I do it?" She just looked at me and smiled and gently nodded her head. I could see it in her eyes and feel it in her calm and solid presence, "Yes, this will work" and "Yes, you can do it" and "No, you will not be having this baby in the OR."

She gave me pep talks that were so encouraging. Her faith fueled me through the moments that I could not fuel myself. Even when I was pushing, I kept asking those questions. At one point she took my hand and put it between my legs and I felt my baby's head! It helped me so much to feel him come down when I pushed. I was overtaken by some kind of superforce as I suddenly understood what to do with my body. It was the only time in my labor I was really able to let go of the doubt in my abilities. As his shoulders were born, I hollered like a madwoman. And I was. I was mad with power and grief and joy and astonishment all at the same time. My midwife lifted my boy right into my arms, looked me in the eyes, and asked me, "Well?"

I remember throwing my head back and taking in a huge breath and looking up at the ceiling while talking out loud, "I did it?" I asked the universe. When I looked back down at him, I knew the truth. It filled my whole body up. I did it.

I have watched the video of his birth and I see what happened after that—the kind of pure joy and that fresh confidence I am oozing. I imagine that is how I looked the first time I got myself across all of the monkey bars at recess in grade school.

—Tammy

Why should I consider an HBAC versus a hospital VBAC?

WHEN CONSIDERING ALL OF the reasons you might want to HBAC, consider all of the reasons any woman would homebirth. They all apply to HBAC mothers. However, there is an additional consideration.

The midwifery model of care is tailor-made for HBAC mothers. Women come to a midwife, sit on her couch, and share their stories. As they are talking, it is also clear that they are seeking. Women who are interested in HBACs often speak about their previous labors in terms of what was missing. They are looking for a new model that is based on respect for their intelligence, maturity, and education. They

The Midwife Says: As you investigate your option to HBAC, you will encounter so much information. Take it all in and then let the pieces come together. After processing everything you hear, learn, experience, and feel, you will get to the answer that is right for you—it is a journey. Don't look for shortcuts. If you run, each step gets you closer to a finish. But each step on a slow walk brings something new into your vision. The HBAC mothers we know have a very broad field of vision. We don't worry about uterine ruptures when we work with HBACs. Our only concern when we come to your home for the birth is how to best support you on the final day of that emotional journey. That's the work of pregnancy and labor for an HBAC mom. That's why you are so special.

have been through the wringer and they know what they *don't* want. Homebirth midwives specialize in translating all of the information from a mother's previous birth experience into mindful attention that addresses their deepest fears and needs.

As for the birth itself, to distinguish between hospital VBACs and HBACs, remove all of the elements they do not have in common. When we take away the uncomfortable continual monitoring (many women do not like the feeling of those tight straps around their belly during labor!), the required IV, the time limits on your length of labor, the internal exams, the environment where you are given a *trial* of labor, and all of the dehumanizing experiences that occur with *any* hospital experience, what are you left with?

You are left with homebirth care: frequent intermittent monitoring with a stethoscope or Doppler (no straps, and you usually don't even need to change position), no IV unless medically necessary, no time limits on the length of your labor (more on that in a moment), internal exams only when you ask for them, an environment where your mid-wife believes that you are in labor (not trying out labor), and unparal-leled support for your unique history and needs.

What is the main characteristic of an HBAC labor?

THE WORK OF AN HBAC labor is different from a standard birth and deserves to be recognized as such; it can be the work of healing from a previous birth experience *and* birthing a new child. That is a lot of work! Healing is meant to take time, sometimes a lot of time. It pulls our fears to us where we first face them, then work through them, and only then can we ease our way past them. While this prepa-ration begins during pregnancy, it is during the labor itself that the long haul of recovery comes to a head.

Because of this, we expect HBAC moms to have very long early labors. Time is an ally, giving them space to be and feel and work. Often, an HBAC labor is like climbing a slab of granite with nothing but sheer determination and bare hands. As these mothers approach the point where their previous labor ended, there can be resistance and fear. The mother may slip back a bit. This is the exact point where a midwife will attach a rope to her and provide the stability for a safe climb. Watching a mother make that climb, tenuous step by tenuous step, we view and treat her with what is known in the psychology world as Unconditional Positive Regard.[1] She is alchemy incarnate, a true miracle in the making. Your HBAC midwife holds a special place of awe for you during these moments and hours.

We don't count or worry about the hours passing, or the sun ris-ing and setting again. Healthy bites of food promote strength for your body while the loving, continuous presence of your team provides an environment of emotional safety. Our words of faith and encourage-ment throughout labor enhance an HBAC mother's subterranean be-lief in herself and her baby. As long as you and Baby are medically safe, the labor is allowed to progress on its own terms and in its own time.

The other thing we have seen a lot of is actually at the complete opposite end of the spectrum. In some labors, especially those where the mother has previously reached full dilation, the body takes on the work itself, and the labor can be very fast. Like a wild chase scene from *The Dukes of Hazzard*, the mind is left in the dust, wondering exactly what just happened. We have seen these women look down at their babies, then look back up at the people around them and ask, *"Is this my baby!?"* and *"What just happened?!"* As the first hours pass, they integrate the events of the body into their mind. Short labors do not mean easy; the intensity of birth is simply compressed. If you receive one of these labors, just know that it is exactly what your baby and your spirit needed.

I've had a c-section. Can I deliver my next baby at home?

MANY THOUSANDS OF WOMEN have done their research and decided that an HBAC is the birth that fits them best. In many states, vaginal births after cesareans are explicitly included in the official scope of practice for midwives. In other states, the right to HBAC is more ambiguous or outright denied. Your local International Cesarean Awareness Network (ICAN) chapter can help you understand your options. We discuss ICAN in detail below.

Is HBAC Safe?

THIS IS A RELATIVE question, of course. What feels dangerous to one practitioner or family may feel perfectly safe to another, as we discussed in our section on perceived risk. There have been some very good studies done on the safety of VBAC, and some very good studies done on the safety of homebirth. Unfortunately, there are very few well-designed studies done on the safety of HBAC. So let's look at the VBAC statistics and see how they apply to homebirth.

The national cesarean rate in the United States is 32.8 percent of all births.[2] This is actually down from 32.9 percent in 2009, the first drop in more than a decade.[3] While we applaud any drop, this is still a deplorable statistic. The World Health Organization suggests that the safe number of c-sections is between 10 and 15 percent.[4] Any more than that, and the surgical risks start to outweigh the benefits. Any lower than that, and true-need surgeries are not being performed.

Almost a third of all births are the result of major surgery; subsequently, there are many women considering VBACs. Some of them are truly traumatized by their experience, while others simply want a different type of birth. Either way, they are led to VBAC, and for some, remembering their previous hospital experience, it is a small jump to homebirth. This is especially true for women who had a cesarean for "failure to progress." For whatever reason, be it physiological, psychological, or emotional, some women simply labor better when they are relatively alone, in their own space, and where they feel most safe. This is normal and healthy! It is a characteristic of all mammals. The wildebeest has to be able to stop laboring and hide if a lion approaches. Our bodies (and our brains are definitely a big part of our bodies) sometimes cannot tell the difference between a lion and an internal fetal monitor. So if this is you, we have great news: you did not "fail" to progress in your labor. Your body actually worked wonderfully. It was providing you with the opportunity to find safety, which is the most important basic element of a healthy birth.

So, are there any hard numbers on HBAC at all?

THERE IS ONE STUDY, by The National Birthday Trust, which included a small piece of the HBAC puzzle.[5] This is the most comprehensive study on homebirth ever recorded in the United Kingdom. It is extraordinarily well designed, and tried to control for almost every variable possible. Planned homebirths were compared with planned hospital births. Even the homebirths that transferred to a hospital still had their data included in the homebirth results. This is very significant. The women in the two groups were matched for age, number of other children, and geography, and significant obstetrical history. Of the 5,971 mothers who planned to birth at home, only 53 of them were planning an HBAC.[6] This is an extremely small number. But of those 53, 38 of them, 72 percent, did have their babies at home without any of the major interventions that come with a hospital birth.[7]

Assuming that the rest of the women who transferred to the hospital had a repeat cesarean (and we do not actually know that; we are just assuming the worst-case scenario for argument's sake), that is a 28 percent c-section rate. That rate is lower than the average American mother walking into a hospital to birth, VBAC or not.

Okay, so what exactly is everyone so afraid of?

THE WICKED WITCH OF the West in this story is *uterine rupture*. This occurs when the uterus opens up, usually (but not necessarily) along the old scar. This sounds superscary, but like most things, if you shine some light in its direction, it either looks better or scurries off under the sink. In this case, it looks a lot better than it sounds.

Uterine ruptures can take two forms. They can be catastrophic, where the uterus comes apart to such an extent that the baby is forced into the abdominal cavity. True catastrophic rupture occurs in .3 to .7 percent of all VBAC labors.[8] *Of these*, 6 percent resulted in perinatal death.[9]

However, uterine ruptures can also be small and have no impact on the pregnancy. These do not require any treatment and are often not even noticed by doctors unless there is an ultrasound during labor or a repeat cesarean. In one study of 17,000 women having VBACs, the minor uterine rupture rate was 1.1 percent.[10] Just for comparison, a first-time mother with no previous uterine scar has a .0015 to .008 chance of uterine rupture.[11]

Statistics for rupture traditionally have not distinguished between the two. They also used to not distinguish between mothers who were induced during their trial of labor after a cesarean (TOLAC), although that has changed in the last several years. One recent study concluded that the rate of uterine rupture among mothers who were not induced, who had had one prior c-section, and whose scar was low and transverse (bikini cut), was 0.7 percent.[12]

What are the maternal and neonatal mortality rates for HBACs?

BECAUSE WE HAVE NO good research showing HBAC neonatal or maternal mortality rates, we have to default to the VBAC numbers:

- VBAC maternal mortality rate: .0038 percent [13]

- Elective repeat cesarean delivery mortality rate: .0134 percent [14]

- VBAC perinatal mortality rate: .013 percent [15]

- Elective repeat cesarean perinatal mortality rate: .005 percent [16]

Can I have an HBAC if I've had more than one cesarean?

WHILE YOU CAN HAVE an HBAC after multiple cesareans (HBAMC), it can be more difficult to find a midwife to attend you. HBAMCs are rarely encouraged by midwifery associations and quite frowned upon by most physicians.

While the American Congress of Obstetricians and Gynecologists (ACOG) does not support HBAMCs, their *Practice Bulletin* from August 2010 states that, "TOLAC [Trial of Labor after Cesarean] may be considered in women with 2 previous low transverse cesarean deliveries." They note that this is based on limited or inconsistent scientific evidence, and it seems to be in response to patient demand. Midwives are facing the same demand, and with informed consent and a high level of parent-led education, some midwives are willing to serve this population.

A 2010 meta-analysis showed that the uterine rupture rate for vaginal births after two or more cesareans was 1.5 percent (about 1 percent higher than it is for one cesarean). This study included inductions and augmentations—both of which carry significantly higher risk of uterine rupture than spontaneous labor.

While there is an increased risk associated with VBAMCs, they may also help women avoid the possible future risks of having multiple cesarean deliveries. These risks include:

- infection
- hysterectomy
- bladder injury
- bowel injury
- transfusion
- abnormal placenta conditions in future pregnancies

If your family plans include many children, please know that the above risks increase exponentially after three cesareans. In many cases, VBAC, regardless of the number of prior uterine surgeries, may be the safest way to go.

I am sure that I want an HBAC but I am really worried it won't work and I will feel like a failure. Is it worth the try?

THE GOAL WITH ANY pregnancy is that when you are holding your baby, regardless of the type of birth that got her into your arms, you will feel that you owned every decision that led to that moment. In hindsight, it is this type of involvement, or the lack of it, that can determine how you feel about your birth. Many HBAC mothers talk about the fear of failure in their stories, and over the course of their pregnancies come to feel that they have really given it their all, regardless of outcome. It is important to note here that an HBAC transfer is not a failure. It is the result of hard and dedicated work and some combination of things that were completely out of your control.

Educating yourself and putting in the physical effort throughout pregnancy takes on a new meaning with HBAC moms. We find them to be uber-dedicated to setting themselves up to do their best. Your midwife will work very hard with you to be aware of all that you are doing along the way. If you do have a repeat cesarean, hopefully it will feel different from the first one. Hopefully you will know with absolute certainty that it was a necessary procedure.

> Overall I feel very good, both physically and emotionally. This is a happy surprise for me. After the birth of my first by c-section, I felt sad for a long time. This time the feelings of sadness are gone. I just feel happy to be with him and really good about all of the work I did to prepare for my birth. My body feels good from laboring—it feels worked and used for the purpose I wanted to use it for. My baby had a role in his birth, and I know he came in the way he needed to.
>
> —Janna

Mothers who have repeat cesareans after a transfer from an HBAC usually need to grieve the loss of their dreams, but the grief is tempered by the bodily knowledge that they have used every resource available to them throughout pregnancy and labor.

Finding an HBAC Midwife

I want to have an HBAC, but I'm having trouble finding a midwife to attend me. Help!

EVEN IN STATES WHERE HBAC is accepted and encouraged, it can still be difficult to find a midwife. Some midwives have read the data and do not feel comfortable with the risk of uterine rupture. Others, who are required by their states to carry malpractice insurance, find that their policies do not cover HBAC. If this is the case, it is impossible for the midwives to get reimbursement from clients' health insurance companies, so it may not make financial sense for them to accept HBAC clients. And sometimes, there are so few midwives that it is just hard to find them at all.

The best place to find an HBAC-friendly midwife is through word of mouth. Ask around in your peer group, especially if you have friends who have had homebirths. Call around to some midwives—they usually know which of their peers work with HBACs. Doulas, perinatal massage therapists, prenatal yoga teachers, and La Leche League leaders often keep a list of midwives for referral purposes. Your local chapter of ICAN can be absolutely invaluable in your search.

You can also ask via different Internet groups, especially those devoted to natural living. Facebook has numerous pages designed to connect mothers to mothers, as do Google+ and other social media. Michelle describes her experience with an HBAC midwife:

> Nothing is more discouraging than to inherently know your capabilities and have no one believe or trust in you. I always knew my body could birth my babies. I did not, however, always recognize that birth was more than just a means to have a baby. Birth is this amazing journey that you and your baby take that is mind-blowingly wonderful when it is allowed to happen without intervention. Done right, it is like being in a cocoon of love created by you and those you have carefully chosen to witness this sacred and holy experience.
>
> I assumed that hospitals were safe places to have babies and doctors and nurses could be trusted to help birth my babies the safest and most efficient way possible. This cost me dearly. My first birth was a scheduled cesarean because my baby was "too big." They preyed on my fear of the "what ifs" and quickly got my compliance by stating "Your baby will die if the shoulder gets stuck." Who is going to argue with that?
>
> In my second pregnancy, I still had hope of a vaginal birth. I took a stand in my thirty-ninth week, canceled my scheduled cesarean (baby was supposedly bigger than my first), and switched to a hospital with nurse-midwives. These midwives offered hope and would allow me to attempt a VBAC. Within minutes of arriving at the hospital, I had a nurse laugh at my insistence on a drug-free birth.
>
> Labor was not progressing quickly enough for them, so my nurse-midwife convinced me a little Pitocin would be okay. I

allowed it and my contractions became so so strong, with no break in between. After enduring this excruciating pain for several hours, I decided on an epidural. My nurse-midwife looked my husband and me in the face and said there were no risks from an epidural. Four hours later, I awoke with heart palpitations. I was told my blood pressure had dropped and was given ephedrine (without my consent) to raise my blood pressure. My baby's heart rate was in the high 170s and it would not go down. After 26 hours of labor, I had an emergency cesarean. "Failure to progress" was written into my chart.

When I became pregnant with my third baby, I knew I could not birth my baby in a hospital. I would not have a third cesarean. I finally came to the realization that if I wanted natural childbirth, I needed a true midwife and a homebirth. The only way to rid your mind of fear is to saturate it with truth. I began to research vaginal birth after multiple cesareans, risk of c-sections versus VBACs, uterine rupture statistics, mortality rates in moms and babies with homebirths and hospital births. I learned the truth about the "so-called" risks of VBACs and learned the real truth of the risk of cesareans and interventions. When I was confident of my decision to birth my baby at home, with faith and patience I began my search for the person who I would allow this privilege.

As I write this, tears are flowing down my face at the memory of the first moment I walked through the door at my midwife's office. I knew the moment I laid my eyes on her that my baby and I were safe. Our birth would be honored. She believed me when I said I believed I could birth my baby. Words cannot adequately describe the feeling of finally having someone agree, without a doubt, with what I already knew.

With each appointment, friendship bloomed between myself, my midwife, and her students. Appointments became more like having tea with girlfriends. I was allowed as much time as I needed to talk through my hopes, fears, and dreams. Most times my appointments were an hour long, with no threat of having to rush through them. I needed those times to build the mental and emotional strength I needed for my birth. I was covered with kisses and my baby was spoken to with such love. My tummy was touched with such care and tenderness. My baby and I were loved through my entire pregnancy.

By the time my labor started, I was excited for birth. I knew I would have the birth I wanted. I labored for a very very long time, and pushed for what seemed like forever. I was loved and encouraged through every contraction. When I was discouraged, each one of those beautiful women encouraged me to continue to fight. They never allowed me to believe I couldn't do this. The moment Elijah James was born, every hope and dream I had about birth was affirmed. I have never experienced a greater joy than that moment.

Two and one half years after Elijah James' birth, Violet Sophia was born exactly as he was, in a candlelit room, surrounded by these amazing women who promise and deliver, literally, your hopes and dreams. They represent what birth is meant to be. I would have been robbed of the two greatest days of my life if I had not found them. I am forever grateful for the lifelong friendships I gained through my births.

—Michelle

Finding Peer Support for HBAC

How can I find other women who have done this?

THE INTERNATIONAL CESAREAN AWARENESS Network (ICAN) is a nonprofit, volunteer-based organization. It provides education and support for cesarean recovery and promotes VBACs. There are 130 ICAN chapters worldwide. There is probably one near you. ICAN chapters have online forums and usually offer in-person meetings on a monthly basis. They provide invaluable support for women who have had a cesarean birth. You will meet women like you as well as doulas and midwives who support VBAC moms. It is incredibly

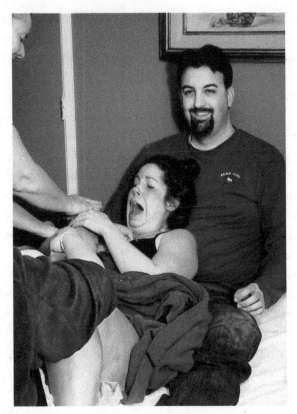

Celebrating an HBAC

powerful to share your story, feelings, and thoughts with others and to hear theirs.

> After my cesarean, I was told by the surgeon, the nurses, and everyone who provided care for me that I should just focus on the fact that I was healthy and that I have a healthy baby. This was offensive to the very core of my soul. I live in America—I never expected to die from childbirth. Telling me that the absolute lowest common denominator was something I should be thankful for was a shock to my system. I struggled with tremendous feelings of guilt and shame from this pressure to concede my values to theirs. It was not until I attended an ICAN

meeting that I came to understand that a safe birth and a good birth can and should be the same birth. For my next pregnancy I found care from a midwife who reaffirmed this and shared my values.

When I went into labor I posted on my ICAN group and asked for good thoughts. Throughout my labor I would check my e-mail for responses. It felt like the whole sisterhood of women was whispering into the wind on my behalf. I could feel them with me on my journey. After my baby was born I was so excited to share the news that I had done it—I had my doula post the good news for me!

—Julie

To locate an ICAN chapter near you, visit http://ican-online.org. Ashley found her midwife through her local chapter. Her story follows.

That night before my birth, I remember crying, cuddling next to my two-year-old, remembering her birth. I had tried so hard to birth her naturally, to have a VBAC. Her older brother had been a surprise footling breech after an easy labor to 8cm at a birth center. I was rushed by ambulance to have a cesarean, even though I was easily at 10cm. It was scary and traumatic. With my daughter, I wanted a VBAC. I envisioned it, I prepared. I was so sure it would be fine. But the labor was very long, very painful, and at a hospital. She was born by a second, very unwanted cesarean. She screamed for hours after her birth, seemingly echoing my own pain.

I was determined that this baby would be born at home, at my midwife's house. I knew that I would not step foot in a hospital again unless it was a true emergency. Every night, before I went to sleep, I imagined myself giving birth. I imagined the baby pushing through me and out, myself unfolding like a rose blooming. I was able to so fully relax and journey into my mind, this became an awesome experience in meditation. And this night, cuddled next to my daughter was different only because

I was remembering her birth—so hard, so cold and full of intervention, so incredibly painful. And I cried, partly out of fear that it would happen again, partly out of remembrance of the emotional and physical pain and sadness.

I dozed off, then awoke again around 11:00 p.m. and found my way to my bed and my sleeping husband. I lay in bed for a while, awake, feeling the heavy baby inside of me. Just as I dozed off, I felt a pop and a gush of warm fluid. I knew that my waters had broken. I found it a bit disconcerting, like something leaving my body that I wasn't sure I wanted to leave.

I got out of bed and went to the bathroom. Definitely leaking fluid. Definitely waters broken. I looked at the time: 11:30 p.m. My thoughts went to the ferry . . . we had to catch one to get to my midwife's house—she had graciously offered us her basement for my birth. The last ferry of the night was at 12:30 a.m. I called my midwife and she told us to come over, "Even if you just hang around. You've done this twice already, you could be fast." I had not had any contractions, but I felt different. My belly felt tighter. I felt slightly uncomfortable. I was nervous.

My husband kicked it into high gear. He opened the garage door, started up our 1986 VW Vanagon, which coughed a bit of gasoline fumes into the air, and ran upstairs to get the kids. I got some pajama pants on, and as he was loading the older child into the backseat, a contraction hit. A big one. I just stopped; silent, and breathing. As we pulled out of our driveway I had another contraction. I looked at the clock on my cell phone. Tony watched me quietly. Not more than three minutes later, I had another contraction. Quick, tight, and painful. I was nervous . . . would we even make it to my midwife's? Should we turn around and have the baby at home on our own? The pains came three minutes apart and were lasting about sixty seconds.

We made the ferry and my contractions got stronger, much more intense and came every minute or two. I was moaning, then yelling, "Wait, baby. Wait, baby. Wait, baby." And pounding my fist on the seat. Every once in a while, a ferry worker would come check on us.

"How's everything going?" they'd say.

"Fine! Just fine!" Tony would answer.

I tried to appear as calm as possible. But right when we arrived at the other side (about a ten-min. ride), I felt myself starting to push. "I'm starting to push, Tony!" I yelled. I was panicked, now. In transition, I realized afterward.

At this point, I feebly informed Tony I was going to lie down on the floor of the van. With a great amount of trouble, I squished myself down on the floor, having to maneuver in between the seats and in front of my two year old's car seat. At that point I re- member thinking I was not in as much pain as I was on the ferry. I was more relaxed, even though I was starting to push my baby out while crammed onto the floor of our van, speeding down the freeway. But it was true, once pushing started I became much more levelheaded and lucid, able to almost control my labor. My body needed to push, but I remembered reading that one can push gently, slowly, in order to ease the baby out. So I did that. I pushed very gently, only enough to satisfy the urge. I could feel the baby's head inside, but I also realized it had a good ways to go. I wasn't going to suddenly push the baby out on the floor of the van. I hoped not, anyway.

Another ten minutes passed with continued questioning from my kids about where we were going. I went inside myself, breath- ing slowly, consciously relaxing my body and my legs, relaxing every part of myself. Time seemed to both slow and speed up at once. Never did the thought cross my mind that I had a scar on my uterus. I just slowed down and let my body work. It took over. It knew what to do.

We pulled up at Sarah's house at about 1:30 a.m.—only two hours after my water had broken.

The moment that Sarah told me the tub was ready, I was up, stripping off my clothes, and literally hopping in the tub. The pleasure and relief from getting in the water was miraculous. I reclined against the side of the tub with my husband behind me. I was incredibly aware, cognizant, and even talkative during this point of the birth. Sarah held up a mirror for me so I could see the baby's head emerging. I very instinctually felt with my hand the baby's head stretching me as I was pushing, and being so surprised that it didn't hurt more. I would feel a contraction coming, bear down and push and moan and sort of "Ssssss" through my teeth, and then relax. I pushed gently and deliberately. Between contractions I would relax back on Tony, or I would say something, usually asking if everything was okay, if the baby was in the right position. Still fear coming up from my second birth, still a bit of me that thought this wasn't really going to happen.

I gave a few more pushes, and Sarah put away the mirror, and put on gloves. My memory of the actual birth, of the moment of my third child's arrival, is fuzzy. The pushing got more intense, and the burning, the "ring of fire," a bit more intense, but still bearable. And then my midwife leaned forward; I felt pressure from her hands, her telling me to push push push, and then a great pain. I screamed, a very primal scream, but not one of fear. Then I felt the amazing sensation of the baby slipping out of me. My midwife was smiling as she placed this small slippery body on my chest.

I remember these things about that glorious moment: the peacefulness of our baby girl, my elation at holding her there, in the tub, the umbilical cord still attached, the placenta not yet out, Sarah reaching over and speaking to her softly and so welcomingly as she examined her and listened to her lungs and heart, myself exclaiming over and over again, "I did it! We did it!" My older children came into the room, and all of us admired the new, tiny, wet baby with superlong fingers and a bald head, just like the others.

When we finally weighed her, after toweling off, tucking ourselves into cozy blankets, admiring the placenta and the first, tentative suckling, eating some peanut butter toast, hearing the soft, admiring conversation of our doula and midwife and children and mother and sister, she was an even 9 pounds. Bigger than my first two babies born by cesarean, and much faster. Just a bit over three hours, from start to finish. For hours, days, after the birth, I was high. I knew that I could and should birth my baby naturally, for myself, for my body, for my baby. There was no other option. The smiles, the warmth, the pride of that moment will live inside me forever.

—Ashley

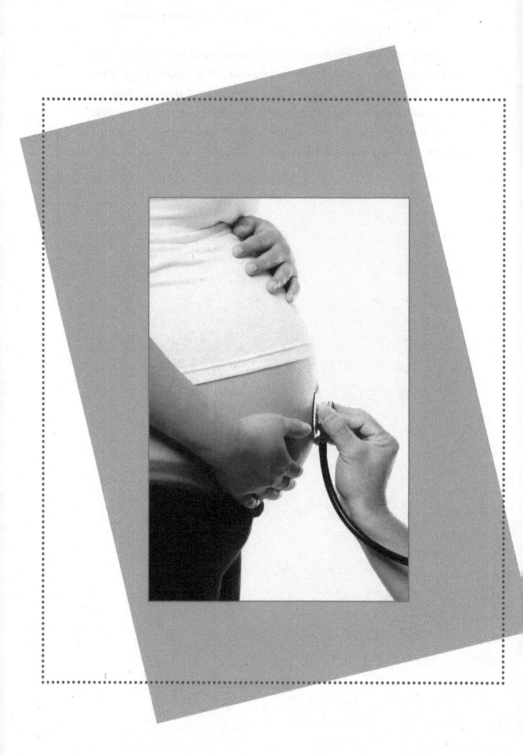

CHAPTER NINE

The Big Ten:
Common Pregnancy-Related Issues

- The emotional experience of pregnancy
- Anemia
- Vitamin D deficiency
- Rhesus factor (aka Rh negative)
- Group beta strep (aka group B strep or GBS)
- Gestational diabetes
- The thyroid
- "I think I'm just plain getting sick. What can I do?"
- Hypertensive disorders
- Miscarriage

MAMA SAYS

The thing about facing down that nutrition demon is that I did it with the support of my midwife. She was relentless in pursuit of my health, she was with me in the fight. In all my years with a doctor, I was never able to understand why it was so important to eat well. But she patiently showed me how what goes in creates who I am in every cell of my body. Then she taught me about food choices. I was able to change my behavior because I finally knew the truth and I had this loving woman telling me, "Here's how it's done, and I'm right here for you while you make these changes."

—Lucy

IN THIS CHAPTER WE are going to tackle The Big Ten. Knowing that it is impossible to write about every topic that will come up in pregnancy, we have chosen to address ten issues that many women experience or ask us about. Every one of these issues can have serious effects on your pregnancy and can affect your and your baby's health and emotional well-being.

Education is great and knowledge is power, which is why we have included this chapter. But we don't want you to be fearful of this information—or any information. The idea is to be aware. Find a good balance between learning enough and yet not becoming overloaded or overwhelmed by the facts. We decided to provide a basic discussion for each topic and to include our own perspective along with good science (when possible). This by no means should replace the discussions you would have with your provider, should you face any of these challenges in your pregnancy.

The Big Ten are The Emotional Experience of Pregnancy, Anemia, Vitamin D Deficiency, Rhesus Factor, Group Beta Strep, Gestational Diabetes, the Thyroid, "I think I'm just plain getting sick. What can I do?," Hypertensive Disorders, and Miscarriage. We hope reading through this section shows you how we approach challenges in pregnancy and birth: the kind of questions we ask, the resources we make use of, and the models for decision making we encourage our mothers to explore.

We know these topics can feel loaded. That is why we highly recommend reading this section or parts of it and then either going for a long walk outside, listening to your favorite music, or just sitting and thinking happy baby thoughts. Let the information settle on the back burner, knowing that if you need it, it is here for you. Know also that if the need arises, you will find meaningful answers from meaningful resources.

Although most of The Big Ten are medical concerns, we will start with your emotional health. Your well-being is the foundation for your physical and spiritual health, and is essential for you to enjoy your pregnancy, your birth, and your baby.

The Emotional Experience of Pregnancy

FIRST OF ALL, WE know you want reassurance that everything is all right. This is perfectly normal. Let us start by saying that for most pregnant women, everything *is* all right—really! Next let us assure you that it is perfectly normal to have thoughts that are at complete odds with one another, or that just make no sense, and for your emotions to flip-flop. Pregnancy is confusing, overwhelming, and mind-blowing. One minute you want to be in control and the next you desperately want someone to tell you what to do. One minute you are despondent because you can no longer reach down to tie your shoes, the next you are overcome with happy tears because you are going to bring forth life. The range of your emotional experiences is wider and deeper than it has ever been before. And as one mom said, "Every experience is felt in three-D." Mothers feel deeply sad at times, giddy and joyful at others, and sometimes each extreme within seconds. This is all common and very, very normal.

Worry is overtaking my life. What should I do?

NO MATTER WHAT SUBJECT we are talking about, expecting moms ask us, "What should I be worried about?" There is a proverb that says, "Worry often gives a small thing a big shadow." Stewing in a broth of all the things that can possibly go wrong during your pregnancy will cast a wide, dark shadow over the entire experience. Worry floods your system with stress hormones, which cross the placenta and course through your baby's bloodstream. We are not sharing this to make you feel guilty—worry and stress are a natural part of life. Your baby will experience these emotions with you just as he will experience the emotions of forgiveness, understanding, and love that naturally follow stressful times.

There are so many changes and issues that can occur during pregnancy. A pregnant woman could run in circles chasing all of the "might be" and "what if" moments that come with this condition! Certainly spending your days reading worst-case or rare scenarios on the Internet is one option for your pregnancy. But to what end? It's better to surround yourself with quality providers and support people who will help you navigate troubled waters should a real problem arise. Having the systems in place to handle each moment as it comes is the most positive maneuver you can make. It allows you to proceed with the health and joy of your pregnancy and let the worries rest.

When it comes to worrying about conditions that occur during pregnancy, we would like to shift the paradigm away from worry and toward one of awareness. Knowing more about your own body and being able to judge when something is wrong is a very important skill for women, particularly pregnant women. While it can be difficult to make this paradigm shift, it is so liberating.

> With my first pregnancy I had very typical, treadmill-like care. I never knew I could question the doctor and decide for myself and my baby which tests I would take. When he ordered a high-level ultrasound (for no reason other than he liked them), I drank my gallon of water and went in for it. I was young and healthy with no significant family history to worry about. I had no reason to suspect there would be any abnormal findings. I received a call that evening from his nurse who curtly told me: "Your baby has Down syndrome." She did not offer any additional information—only suggested I speak to a genetic counselor so that I could prepare.
>
> I spent the week in despair and then I began to notice people with Down syndrome. I fell in love with each of them, from across the street or on the train or in the grocery store. While I realized my capacity to love my child existed regardless of who he or she might be genetically, I cannot say that this eased my worries. Did I do something wrong? Should I be doing something different for the next nearly five months of my pregnancy?
>
> I finally got to meet the genetic counselor who explained to us that the diagnosis was not positive. I had been screened

but not tested. Furthermore, my HMO was in a major American inner-city where thresholds at the lab did not necessarily represent my particular risk levels. When we looked at numbers for areas in the country that were more representative of who I am, the odds that my child had Down's were very unlikely. I should have been relieved, but I was not. I felt compelled to prepare, I grieved over the shift in expectation, and I worried about future children. It was not until I saw my healthy boy that I could at all face what the stress and worry of those months did to us. And then I grieved for spending those days in stress! It took some time to forgive myself and to be able to tell my baby how sorry I was that he gestated in all of that fear.

With the next pregnancy, I got myself to a great midwife, learned to ask a lot of questions, and I went without the tests that had high false-positive rates. I did not opt for ignorance but I did not let potential worry anywhere near me. If real worries crept up, I had a great midwife who did not mind helping me research and discuss until I felt comfortable. I spent time each morning and each evening quietly smiling and thinking about how healthy we were.

When I think back on that first pregnancy, I feel robbed of time I should have had and also grateful—I was forced to take a hard look at my own potential, I made a lot of mistakes, and I became a better mom because of them. I wouldn't recommend learning the hard way if you don't absolutely have to—worry significantly impacts the potential that pregnancy has to bring out health and happiness.

—Carolyn

If you need something to do instead of worrying, pay attention to the health in your body and your baby, and then celebrate it. We encourage you to head downtown or to a busy mall and to look around. Most of the people you see were born healthy—the odds are with you! Embrace your growing belly. Trust your baby. Trust your emotional and physical capabilities.

Some days it feels as if time is standing still, and it is freaking me out. Is it normal to be aware of every single minute of my pregnancy?

THERE MAY BE SEVERAL answers to this. We discuss this in the prenatal chapter when we talk about *chronos* and *kairos* time. Your body is taking you on a journey that is not bound by the second hand of the clock. Mothers often want to just sit and experience what they are feeling. At the same time, the modern world calls. Not many of us can just stop showing up to work and spend our time walking through the Highland heather. Perhaps the tension between everything your body is telling you to do and what you are actually doing with your time increases your awareness of it.

Furthermore, in the same way that your baby's cells are dividing constantly and pushing forward with growth, pregnancy divides and grows mothers. It can feel as though your soul is literally opening and expanding as you gain a new understanding of *life*. This is huge work and is certainly not able to be contained by minutes or hours. Take some time each day to nurture yourself by sitting with these new experiences, if that is what you are called to do.

I know it sounds rude but I am totally selfish right now, and I feel guilty for thinking so much about me!

WE BELIEVE THAT MANY theories about the survival of the species could be taken off the table if any of these scientists would spend time with pregnant women—arguably the most selfish subset of humans we've ever known! While the typical three year old takes a close second, a pregnant mother's focus on herself is actually a focus on all of life's most fundamental issues: How will I keep this baby alive? How will I keep myself alive so that I can nourish and care for her? How can I do all of that really well? Is it wrong to get a pedicure and a massage on the same day?

Before you are overcome with guilt, take a step back and notice the value in these questions. Your focus on yourself is actually the manifestation of an intuitive need to guard your unborn baby by nurturing yourself.

It is common to want to talk about yourself and the pregnancy—a lot. Pregnancy and birth are not experienced separately by the mind and body. They are meant to be felt, regarded, thought about, discussed, and reflected upon.

Major life events, and especially bodily ones such as pregnancy and birth, will alter us in significant degrees if we are open to the experience. Missed opportunities in these areas are missed chances for human spiritual growth. We are meant to experience these events and to be changed by them. Consider your "selfishness" a window into the *self*. It is an opportunity to create new inner dimensions that you will carry forward with you as a partner, friend, and mother.

Sometimes I feel like my emotions, both positive and negative, are too extreme. How can I get them under control?

IT'S SO HARD, ISN'T it? One minute you're Mother Teresa and the next you're Darth Vader. But what if you didn't have to get them under control? What if you just felt them fully? What if you let yourself feel them as deeply as you could, instead? Does that seem scary?

We aren't used to giving our emotions free rein. We're used to reining them in, but this can sometimes cause more problems than if we welcomed them in and accepted them without judgment. Your emotions are a part of you, and you are wonderful. When you feel these strong emotions, instead of pushing them away, do the opposite. Inflate them as big as you can. Really go for it. Take at least a minute, but more is even better. Don't back away. You have the courage you need to do this. And then notice how your body feels. Are your shoulders up around your ears? Are your lips pursed? Is your jaw tight? How is your body interacting with your feelings?

Now slowly, so your emotions don't notice, correct those physical imbalances. Drop your shoulders, relax your lips, and shake out your jaw. Address whatever your body has told you to do. Now bring your awareness back to your emotions. Most likely they will have subsided a bit, even though you gave them more attention and did not shut them down. Repeat the process as needed.

This is soul work, so it's not meant to be easy. And that's okay. You are worth it.

> **The Midwife Says:** We like to do this exercise with our clients: Pull up your sleeve, look at your arm, and flex your biceps hard for thirty seconds and then release them. How does that feel? Now look at your arm again. Where are your muscles?
>
> Our emotions work the same way. We can flex them and pay attention to them or just be aware of them as they arise. Then, when we release that tension, they are still there, only somehow calmer. Letting ourselves really feel our emotions doesn't mean we are necessarily overtaken by them. It just allows us to see them. And then we exhale, and something releases. The emotions, just like the muscles, actually feel better after they get to come out and play.

Anemia

ANEMIA IS VERY COMMON during pregnancy. It can be caused by an iron or a vitamin deficiency, inherited, due to faulty mechanisms in the bone marrow, or can occur as a symptom of a chronic or acute disease. Although there are many types of anemias, if you are pregnant and your body is anemic, it is likely due to iron deficiency in your diet. Therefore, our primary focus in this book is on iron-deficiency anemia. If you have a more complex anemia, or wish to learn more in depth about anemia, we recommend the book *Understanding Anemia* by Ed Uthman, MD.

What is anemia?

ANEMIA COMES FROM THE Greek meaning "without blood." Most of us hear the term "anemia" long before we ever become pregnant. Anemia occurs when there is a decrease in the amount or the size of red blood cells present in your body, and is indicated by red blood cells that look or act abnormally. Anemic red blood cells can appear too light in color, too small or too big, or they can be misshapen. They can even clot together abnormally.

Why is iron deficiency common during pregnancy?

DURING PREGNANCY YOUR BLOOD volume will increase by around 50 percent. This is necessary to address all of the oxygen needs of your pregnant body and to provide oxygen to your baby. As your blood volume expands, your body has to make enough red blood cells to keep up with the new demands. If there is not enough iron in your body to help it generate all of these new red blood cells, you are considered *iron deficient*.

How does iron work in my body?

IRON PROVIDES STABILITY BETWEEN oxygen and hemoglobin. Hemoglobin is the suitcase in which oxygen travels around the body. Iron is like a great baggage handler—it allows the suitcase to hold the oxygen in just the right way so that it gets to the destination on time and in one piece.

In addition to giving our bodies the oxygen we need for good health, iron also allows for the production of red blood cells in the bone marrow.

A Few Cool Red Blood Cell Factoids

- There are 25 trillion red blood cells in our bodies.

- Every second, more than two million new red blood cells are produced by the marrow.

- Red blood cells have a life span of 120 days.

- The function of hemoglobin is to carry oxygen to the entire body.

- The only function of red blood cells is to care for and transport hemoglobin and the oxygen they carry.

What symptoms will I feel if I have iron deficiency anemia?

IF YOU ARE ANEMIC, you will likely feel one or more of the symptoms below. Be sure to tell your midwife if you have any of the following:

- FATIGUE: as the tissues are deprived of oxygen, you will feel exhausted and sleep does not help you recover.

- SHORTNESS OF BREATH WITH EXERCISE OR EXERTION: breathing becomes deeper in an effort to get more oxygen since there are not enough red blood cells to deliver the amount of oxygen needed. This feels like shortness of breath or the inability to "catch your breath."

- PALLOR: an anemic person can appear pale because the blood is being diverted away from the skin and toward the vital organs and systems for the body.

- PICA: this is the compulsion to chew on nonfood items, but especially an overwhelming need to chew ice.

- RAPID HEART RATE: the heart works overtime to try to get more blood to the body.

- RINGING IN THE EARS OR A CONSTANT BUZZING SOUND: this is caused either by oxygen starvation or the rushing of blood through the vessels near the ear at such an increased rate that one "hears" the sound of it.

- SEVERE SYMPTOMS: if your body works too hard to compensate and pulls too much water from other organs to feed the bloodstream, there is a tipping point where the load is too much to handle. In these cases severe symptoms can arise, including dimmed vision (not enough oxygen to the brain), fainting, swelling of the ankles and lower back, pulmonary edema (swelling of your lungs), and heart failure.

How can I get enough iron?

THE ONLY NATURAL WAY that the body can get iron is through diet, where it is absorbed in the upper intestine. If there is excess iron, it is excreted in the feces. Your midwife will probably recommend that you take a supplement, as well as add iron-rich food sources to your diet. Here are the options we recommend:

- Supplements
  - *Florodix Floravital Iron + Herbs (available at flora health.com)* in combination with
  - *Hyland's #4 ferrum phos cell salt tablets (dissolve 16 tablets in a glass of water daily)*
  - *Ask your midwife for a supplement she prefers.*
  - *In severe cases, IV iron therapy may prove useful.*
- Foods Rich in Iron
  - *spinach, broccoli, kale and other dark green leafy vegetables*

- *liver and other meats*

- *poultry (dark meat)*

- *dried fruits (apricots, prunes, figs, raisins, dates)*

- *blackstrap molasses*

- *black beans*

- *nuts and seeds*

- *steel-cut oatmeal*

- *baked potato with skin (in moderation, these potatoes are high on the glycemic index)*

Are there other types of anemia that pregnant women are at risk for?

THERE ARE TWO. THE first is due to folate deficiency and the second, due to B_{12} deficiency. A deficiency of either of these vitamins stalls the production of red blood cells in the bone marrow, causing anemia.

Your midwife can use blood tests to get to the bottom of exactly which type of anemia you have. She can either design a treatment plan for you or refer you to a specialist for further evaluation and care.

Can I still have a homebirth if I have anemia?

THE ANSWER TO THIS will depend upon how anemic you are and what your midwife says. If you are very anemic, you are more susceptible to postpartum hemorrhage.[1] You need to be in a location and with a provider who is comfortable managing postpartum hemorrhage and has the medicine (which may be allopathic or herbal) to do so.

How does anemia affect my baby?

SEVERELY ANEMIC BABIES MAY have worrisome heart rate patterns before they are born. Just like you, your baby needs enough healthy red blood cells to carry oxygen to his entire body. Babies develop quickly—their cells are multiplying every single minute—and they need fuel, in the right composition, to handle this rapid growth effectively.

Breast-fed babies born to vegan mothers are particularly at risk for vitamin B_{12} deficiency, which leads to severe megaloblastic anemia (a type of anemia where the cells are too large) and may cause permanent brain damage. Ideally, vegetarian and vegan mothers will seek counseling from qualified nutritionists who are specially trained in the nutrition of pregnancy.

Babies born to women who remain iron deficient during pregnancy are at increased risk for iron deficiency during the first year of life. These babies tend to have reduced iron stores as well as lower mental and developmental scores over the course of the first year.

Because anemia increases your chances for a postpartum hemorrhage, your risk of postpartum anemia also rises. Mothers with postpartum anemia have a higher risk of postpartum depression, an illness which affects both Mother and Baby.[2]

Working hard to correct problems with anemia during pregnancy pays off in spades for the health of your developing fetus and newborn baby (and of course, you!).

The Body's Ability to Compensate

Through understanding anemia, we can discover some amazing facts about the human body. We learn that when one system is not quite up to par, it will borrow from other systems to compensate for any deficiencies. In the case of anemia, the body will actually redirect the use of oxygen away from the skin and other organs so that the heart and brain remain supported. We also see that what may look like disease can have a higher purpose. In the case of sickle-cell anemia, the particular shape and texture of the cells provides complete immunity from a deadly form of malaria that is common in certain tropical areas. People whose families descend from these areas are most at risk for sickle-cell anemia. Because the malaria is more deadly than the anemia, it makes sense that the body allows this trade-off. The body constantly seeks and adapts in favor of health. If your body is able to adjust this much on its own, imagine what it can do when fully supported through a healthy lifestyle!

Vitamin D Deficiency

THERE IS A PLETHORA of newly published research and revelations about the extensive role that vitamin D plays during pregnancy for both maternal and fetal health. If you are a science-geek (like us!), this is a hot item to watch. Information is pouring out of labs about the exact nature, mechanisms, and function of vitamin D. For example, the Human Genome Project demonstrated that vitamin D is responsible for regulating more than 10 percent of our genes. It strengthens bones, modulates our immune systems, and regulates cell multiplication throughout our bodies. Optimal levels of vitamin D protect us from some cancers, promote breast health, and can even affect our oral health. Thanks to recent research, we now know what the blood levels of vitamin D should be for optimal health in pregnancy and breastfeeding.

Research has shown that an overwhelming number of pregnant women are vitamin D deficient in the United States and worldwide.

Because vitamin D affects a multitude of systems throughout the body, vitamin D deficiency can have negative ramifications for your health and your baby's health. Luckily it is easy to find out what your vitamin D level is—testing is simple and accessible. Increasing the amount in your body is possible through affordable and readily available supplements.

What is vitamin D and how do I get it?

HERE IS A COOL yet confounding fact. Vitamin D is not technically a vitamin, but a hormone that is produced by your body when your skin is exposed to ultraviolet light (the sun).[3] Humans were clearly designed to integrate vitamin D into our systems through sun exposure. One half hour outside on a sunny day, with arms and legs exposed, provides between 10,000 IUs and 25,000 IUs of vitamin D.

Our nutritional options pale in comparison (pun intended!). Vitamin D can be obtained from food and supplements, but most food choices provide only 250 to 500 IUs per serving.

Vitamin D is fat soluble, which means that it is stored in your fat, and too much of it can be toxic. (Most vitamins are water soluble, so if you get more than you need, the excess is excreted through your urine.) Toxicity is extremely rare, though, especially in pregnant women. The amount required every day to maintain and support the development of the baby far exceeds what most women have stored in their bodies or get through their diet while pregnant.

Interestingly, when you get your vitamin D from the sun, the body has a failsafe mechanism built in to keep you from producing too much. You only have to worry about toxicity if you take supplements.

What are the effects of vitamin D deficiency on my pregnancy?

VITAMIN D DEFICIENCY HAS been linked to an increased risk of cesareans, preeclampsia, gestational diabetes, and bacterial vaginosis.[4]

Multiple studies have shown that there is a link between low vitamin D levels and periodontal disease.[5] This is important because periodontal disease in pregnancy is directly associated with adverse pregnancy outcomes.

Vitamin D promotes calcium absorption in the gut, which is important not only for bone health but also for prevention of preeclampsia. In fact, if your blood pressure is high, your midwife will likely look at vitamin D and calcium supplementation as part of the initial treatment plan.

Additionally, many mothers feel pain in their muscles, joints, and bones during pregnancy. While there are many causes for this kind of pain, researchers have found that vitamin D in combination with physical therapy and painkillers (when necessary) plays a significant role in alleviating the pain.[6]

What are the effects of vitamin D deficiency on my baby?

VITAMIN D DEFICIENCY HAS been linked to low birth weight, neonatal rickets, a risk of neonatal hypocalcemia, asthma, and type 1 diabetes.[7] Poor postnatal growth, bone fragility, and increased incidence of autoimmune diseases have been linked to low vitamin D levels during pregnancy and infancy.[8]

A multiyear study evaluated nine year olds for several factors and linked their mother's low vitamin D levels late in pregnancy to significantly lower whole body and lumbar spine bone mineral content when compared to children whose mothers had higher blood levels of vitamin D during pregnancy.[9]

How do I know if I have enough vitamin D?

WE RELY ON THE recommendations of the Vitamin D Council (www.vitamindcouncil.org), a nonprofit organization that connects the most recent peer-reviewed research on vitamin D with providers and consumers. They recommend that pregnant women maintain blood serum levels between 50 and 80 ng/ml. Your midwife can take a simple blood test to measure your vitamin D levels. If your initial blood work is below or on the lower end of that range, begin a program to increase it and have your midwife retest you at your next appointment.

What foods are good sources of vitamin D?

HERE ARE A FEW samples measured in international units (IUs):

- cod liver oil (1 teaspoon): 400
- canned wild salmon (3 ounces): 530
- Silk brand light plain soymilk (one serving): 338
- orange juice from concentrate fortified with vitamin D (one serving): 259
- nonfat milk (one serving): 246

Several processed foods, such as cereals, have vitamin D infused into them but we prefer to focus on options that don't come packaged in sugar. As you can see, compared with sunlight or supplements, food sources are not our best sources for vitamin D.

What kind of supplements should I take and in what dose?

YOUR MIDWIFE WILL LIKELY have a brand of vitamin D that she prefers. It can come in varying strengths of capsules or in liquid form. Regardless of the brand or strength, you want to take vitamin D_3 (cholecalciferol). This is the most bioavailable form of vitamin D. This is especially important in Northern climes, with even less sunlight.

Professor Bruce Hollis, MD, a leading expert in vitamin D, and his colleague Carol L. Wagner, MD, recently completed a National

Institutes of Health study on pregnancy and vitamin D.[10] They were trying to understand how effective different doses are at maintaining vitamin D levels for pregnant and lactating women. There were nearly five hundred women of various ethnicities enrolled over four years. The mothers were divided into three groups and given different dosages. The control group took a dose of 400 IU, the recommended daily allowance (RDA), the second group took 2,000 IU, and the third group took 4,000 IU of vitamin D (ten times the RDA). At 12 weeks gestation, each mother began taking their assigned amount and continued to take this dosage throughout their pregnancy.

The results of the study showed conclusively that pregnant women need 4,000 IU daily and lactating women need 6,400 IU daily in order to maintain vitamin D levels high enough to meet the demands of their expectant and nursing bodies.

Many women will find that they need higher amounts than this to maintain healthy levels. Clinically obese women absorb less vitamin D than their thinner counterparts do, and will need to take higher-than-recommended doses.[11] The best way to know how much you should be taking is to test your levels once per month and adjust accordingly as your pregnancy advances.

I love to be in the sun but I always wear sunscreen; will I still get vitamin D when I am outside?

NO. USING A SUNSCREEN with as little as a 15-factor protection cuts the skin's vitamin D production by 99 percent, rendering the sun ineffective as a source of vitamin D.[12]

We are not promoting risking skin cancer in this book, but we believe that there is a sweet spot between under- and overexposure. A simple way to get that healthy exposure is to go for a walk outside, head to the beach, or just lounge on your deck in the sun for 10 to 30 minutes per day (depending on the strength of the sun) with no sunscreen on. Use your judgment to avoid getting burned, and maintain a diet high in omega-3s, which will help your skin stay healthy.

Rhesus Factor (aka Rh Negative)

YOU WILL LIKELY HEAR the term "Rh negative" or "Rh positive" when your midwife is reviewing your initial blood work. It is actually written out *Rh-negative* or *Rh-positive*, but we will use the simplified "Rh negative" since that is the terminology your midwife will use. Regardless of the technical-speak, we are here to discuss the presence or absence of a protein called Rhesus (Rh) that is found on the surface of your red blood cells. About 15 percent of the population in America do not have the Rhesus factor and are therefore considered Rh negative. If you fall into this group, you will need to make specific care decisions during your pregnancy and after the birth.

Why is it a problem if my blood is Rh negative?

YOUR IMMUNE SYSTEM IS designed to create antibodies when it comes in contact with something that could compromise your health, like bacteria or a virus. Antibodies are very good at what they are designed to do: attack foreign intruders in your bloodsteam. For example, if your immune system is working properly, it attacks the cold virus and renders it harmless so that you don't get sick. In these cases, antibodies are a good thing.

If, on the other hand, your Rh negative blood and your baby's Rh positive blood mix, it is a different story. Your immune system will create antibodies designed to kill any Rh positive red blood cells they encounter.

While this isn't a problem for the first pregnancy that it occurs with, it is a problem for subsequent pregnancies *if that baby is Rh positive also.* Why? Remember the antibodies that your body created to destroy any Rh positive cells? They stay in your bloodstream for life. So when you are pregnant with your second or later babies, and those babies are Rh positive, your antibodies will recognize your baby's blood cells as foreign invaders and attack them.

The resulting destruction of red blood cells can cause your baby to become ill. This condition is known as hemolytic disease of the newborn. Without treatment it can cause anemia, jaundice, brain damage, and heart failure in the baby.

The Midwife Says: Rh antibodies are just like a virus, bacteria, or organ transplant: the body's immune system wants to protect you from anything that does not seem to belong. With this in mind, it seems that any pregnancy would be recognized as foreign and attacked when the placenta begins to attach to the uterine wall. It is an incredible testament to the sophisticated adjustments the pregnant body makes from the moment of conception that the placenta and baby are nourished and not expelled!

Hold up! How can my blood mix with my baby's? I thought we had two different systems?

YOU ARE CORRECT. YOUR bloodstream is separate from your baby's. They can, however, mix under certain conditions:

- a miscarriage or abortion
- an ectopic pregnancy
- a fall or other accident that affects the abdomen (such as a car accident)
- a placental abruption (even a minor one)
- uterine bleeding of unknown origins

You mentioned treatment—should I be treated or should my baby be treated, and if so, how?

THERE ARE TREATMENTS FOR both mothers and babies.

For You

- If you are Rh negative, you will be offered medication called Rh immune-globulin (RhoGAM) at around 28 weeks of pregnancy.

- You will be offered it again within seventy-two hours after birth *if your baby is Rh positive* (blood from your baby's cord will be sent to the lab immediately after birth to determine her Rh status) so that if your blood mixed with hers you will not develop antibodies.

- RhoGAM works like a vaccine and will prevent your body from producing any antibodies even if your baby's blood mixes with yours.

- You will also be offered RhoGAM during your pregnancy if you experience a fall, accident, any bleeding, or if you have any invasive procedures such as an amniocentesis.

For Your Baby

- If your blood test shows that you have developed antibodies and are currently pregnant, the baby will be monitored closely.

- If your antibodies are killing the baby's red blood cells too quickly, your baby will receive blood transfusions while it is still en utero or just after delivery. These transfusions exchange the baby's Rh positive blood for Rh negative blood. The antibodies stop destroying your baby's red blood cells and she can continue to grow and develop.

How effective are these treatments?

SINCE THE ADVENT OF routine treatment of at-risk women, incidence of Rh sensitization (women who carry the antibodies) has declined from 45 cases per 10,000 births to 10.2 cases per 10,000 births, with less than 10 percent requiring intrauterine transfusion.[13]

Before any interventions were available, the perinatal mortality rate for newborns with hemolytic disease was 50 percent. With treatment, that number is down to 16 percent.[14]

Tell me about RhoGAM. Does it have any side effects?

THE INITIAL RHOGAM SHOT was developed by Ortho-Clinical Diagnostics, part of Johnson and Johnson, and was first administered to a New Jersey woman in 1968.[15] RhoGAM is a human blood product. Steps are taken during the manufacturing process to eliminate any pathogens, but, of course, the risk can never be absolutely zero. If you belong to a religious group that traditionally refuses blood products, please have a discussion with your spiritual advisor before making any decisions.

As with any injection, there is a chance of swelling and infection, as well as rare allergic reactions.

Are there any reasons not to take the RhoGAM treatment?

ONE OF THE RISKS is the lack of risk. There is conflicting data on how many pregnant women actually experience any mixing of their blood with their unborn baby's, outside of a traumatic event. In the cases we have mentioned where the blood can mix, the course of care is very clearly in favor of receiving the medicine.

If you would like to understand the history, uses, and risks of RhoGAM in greater depth, we recommend reading *Anti-D in Mid-*

wifery: Panacea or Paradox? by Sara Wickham, RM, MA, BA (Hons), PGCE(A).

If I refuse testing or treatment, how will I know if my baby gets sick?

YOUR BABY MAY EXPERIENCE jaundice, lethargy, and low muscle tone if the symptoms are mild. For mild Rh incompatibility, babies are usually treated with breastfeeding and phototherapy using bilirubin lights.

More severe cases can cause brain damage, fluid buildup and swelling in the baby, seizures, and problems with mental function, movement, hearing, and speech.[16] Severe incompatibility can be fatal.

Group Beta Strep
(aka Group B Strep or GBS)

GROUP BETA STREP (GBS) is just one of many types of bacteria that normally live in our bodies. GBS is not a sexually transmitted disease—it is perfectly natural and cannot be controlled by a person's behavior or cleanliness.

Since GBS is in "The Big Ten" chapter, and there are a lot of words on the next few pages, there must be something more to it than that, right? The trouble with GBS comes into play when there is an over-colonization of it in the vagina and/or rectum.

As she is born, your baby may be exposed to GBS in the birth canal and potentially become ill. There are simple tests to check for colonization and some options for treatment plans. Many parents struggle with GBS testing and treatment because on the one hand, the likelihood of their baby getting an infection is pretty small if they do not have any risk factors. On the other hand, if the baby does get a GBS infection, it can be life threatening.

What is GBS?

GBS IS A NATURALLY occurring bacteria found in the throat, intestines, and vagina of pregnant and nonpregnant women. GBS is migratory; it comes and goes depending on the flora in your digestive tract. You may test positive one day, and negative another. You may be negative during one pregnancy, and positive with the next. Regardless of the potential for change, most providers test only one time and consider those results valid for five weeks.

If it's so normal, why the big to-do?

THE FEAR WITH GBS is that during birth, your baby will come into direct contact with the bacteria and she will get an infection. GBS is the leading cause of pneumonia, blood infections, and meningitis in newborns.[17]

When do I take the test?

WOMEN OFTEN WONDER BOTH why we are testing for something that may or may not be there when they give birth and why we don't just test during labor. The short answer is that we are doing the best we can with the technology we have to get the information we need to try to prevent neonatal deaths from GBS infections. Until tests are readily and cheaply available that give quick results and can be used during labor, this test will be offered between 35 and 37 weeks.

How do I take the GBS test?

THE TEST IS EASY and painless. You or your midwife will simply take a sample from your vagina and rectum using a long swab.

I tested positive for GBS. What does this mean?

ABOUT 25 PERCENT OF healthy pregnant women test positive for significant GBS colonization. You will not feel sick or show any other symptoms normally associated with bacterial overload. It simply means that you have a level of colonization in your vagina and/or rectum that merits talking about potential treatments and outcomes.

I tested positive at 37 weeks, but could I be negative when I give birth?

YES. THIS IS ONE of the factors that make GBS testing and treatment so frustrating. If the GBS levels go back down but you do not know it, you will receive antibiotics for absolutely no reason.

This is a concern for many people who worry about building antibiotic resistance in themselves and their babies. During the past decade, while GBS infections have decreased due to the routine use of antibiotics, other newborn infections, especially E. coli, have risen.[18] E. coli is very resistant to the standard course of antibiotics, making it difficult to treat. In one study, done in 2002, researchers looked at 70 premature babies, born over a two-year period, who were infected with E. coli. Among them, 29 percent had bacteria resistant to ampicillin in 1998, while by 2000, the number had jumped to 80 percent.[19]

Under normal circumstances, babies are colonized with their mother's beneficial bacteria. Antibiotics disrupt this process. This increases your baby's risk of gastrointestinal distress and disease, allergies, and asthma, among other long-term health effects.

I tested negative at 37 weeks, but could I be positive when I give birth and put my baby at risk?

YES. WE STRONGLY RECOMMEND preventative action to help control GBS regardless of the results of your 37-week test. Both of the methods we like, discussed below, add to your overall health regardless of your GBS status.

What are some natural, preventative methods for keeping GBS colonization in check?

WE'RE SO GLAD YOU asked. As we're fond of saying, the best defense is a great offense. There are two great proactive natural methods to try:

- Take a daily probiotic to keep your digestive flora balanced. You should take these throughout pregnancy and while nursing.

- Eat raw garlic. Garlic is a powerful antibiotic that has been shown to kill GBS.[20] It also leaves behind a powerful odor, so have your partner join in your culinary activities—two people smelling like garlic is better than one, for preserving the peace! The active antimicrobial ingredient in garlic is *allicin*. It is released upon cutting or crushing the clove. It may not entirely eliminate the GBS in your body but it can reduce the level of colonization.

    - *Slice it raw into your salads.*

    - *Make fresh garlic hummus.*

    - *Chop up a clove and mix it with a teaspoon of honey, then swallow it without chewing.*

    - *Place a peeled, halved clove between your toes for two hours or overnight.*

    - *Place a peeled, halved clove into your vagina for two hours or overnight. You can use a needle and thread to make a tamponlike string for easy removal. This delivers antibiotic powers straight to the source. Using this protocol for two nights on, one night off for 15 days before your test and again 15 days before your due date can get the levels down.*

You say that most women have some GBS, but most babies do not get sick. How is this possible?

HAPPILY, YOU PROVIDE A lot of immunity for your baby against GBS and a variety of other infections. Most mothers have immunity to the GBS strains that live in their birth canal (which is why they do not get urinary tract infections from its presence).

Your antibodies are transferred across the placenta to your baby around 32 weeks of pregnancy, which is why your baby's own immune system can usually cope with any GBS exposure.

I have tested positive; what is the likelihood that my baby will get an infection?

ACCORDING TO THE CENTERS for Disease Control and Prevention,

- one in 4,000 if you test positive and receive antibiotics
- one in 200 if you test positive, do not receive antibiotics, and have no other risk factors
- one in 25 if you test positive, do not receive antibiotics, and have other risk factors

Four to six percent of babies who become ill due to GBS will die.[21]

It is important for homebirth parents to know that the incidence of GBS in newborns is based upon research done in large hospitals that care for high-risk mothers. These facilities routinely have procedures that homebirth midwives do not, including the following:

- MANY VAGINAL INTERVENTIONS (from regular vaginal exams, to probes and lines that are pushed into the vagina, to rupturing the membranes prior to birth), which all increase the risk that the baby will be exposed to GBS even before the birth as the bacteria can travel up with the instrument, equipment, or hand, into the amniotic fluid and flourish there)

- CONTROLLED DELIVERY OF THE BABY (if your provider stops the natural progress or alters the natural direction of a birthing baby, he can inadvertently expose the baby's nose and mouth to the amniotic fluid that comes just behind it; this fluid picks up GBS as it runs down the vagina and out of the body—and if it rushes over the baby's face, the baby can become infected)

I have tested positive and understand that other issues may increase the chances of my baby getting sick. What are they?

YOUR BABY HAS A higher risk of developing a GBS infection if

- you have a previous baby who developed a GBS infection
- your baby is born before 32 weeks of gestation
- your water is broken longer than 18 hours before your baby is born
- you develop a fever during labor
- you have a urinary tract infection during pregnancy that was cultured and shown to be caused by GBS

I do want to take antibiotics but the thought of an IV really terrifies me. Can I take a course of oral antibiotics before labor begins?

NO. ORAL ANTIBIOTICS ARE not known to be effective against GBS.

I really don't like antibiotics. Are there any alternatives?

YES. CHLORHEXIDINE (KNOWN AS Hibiclens) is popular among some homebirthers instead of antibiotics. It is used in a douche at regular intervals throughout labor. Mothers simply stand in the shower and use the douche vaginally. More and more midwives are offering this as a viable treatment during labor, as more and more research shows that it is an effective alternative. One large, well-designed study from Italy showed that chlorhexidine and ampicillin had the same efficacy in preventing newborn GBS, and that the chlorhexidine group had a lower incidence of E. coli.[22]

The CDC does not support the use of Hibiclens. They recommend that all women who test positive receive IV antibiotics at regular intervals throughout labor.[23] Additionally, the use of Hibiclens can alter the flora in your vagina, so it is important to talk to your midwife about how to restore balance during the postpartum period.

I have tested positive; can I still birth at home with GBS?

EACH MIDWIFE WILL HAVE her own answer to this question. Some midwives are not allowed to carry or administer IV antibiotics. If she is comfortable with it, Hibiclens can be used instead. You also have the right to refuse any treatment, and many women do. Ask your midwife to share her protocols and thoughts regarding GBS.

I tested positive and plan on using Hibiclens. How will I know if my baby develops a GBS infection?

TAKE A DEEP BREATH. The good news is that the likelihood is very, very high that you will be aware of and will observe your baby starting the first minute she is born and continuing until some eighteen years or longer into the future. Homebirth parents tend to observe their babies closely, and it would be rare for them to miss signs of infection. (If you do find yourself overwhelmed and feel you are not providing good care for your baby, call your midwife, physician, or a family member and ask for help.)

Specifically, symptoms of GBS infection in a baby include these:

- difficulty breathing
- fever or abnormally low body temperature
- jaundice
- poor feeding
- vomiting
- seizures
- swelling of the abdomen
- bloody stools

Otherwise, here's the thing about sick babies: babies who are sick, look sick. They act lethargic and do not nurse well. Their playfulness diminishes or stops. Their temperature will drop or rise (a low temperature can be a sign of infection in a newborn). They do not pee and poop as much as they do when they are healthy.

If your baby stops acting like herself, either emotionally or physically, call your midwife or pediatrician. Providers expect these calls from new parents and should respond to your instincts with support. Never be shy about following your gut, even when you don't have concrete evidence that something is wrong. If there is something wrong, then you have placed your baby in the right hands for further care. If everything is fine, you will feel reassured and able to move forward. Seems like a win-win to us.

Gestational Diabetes

WHILE THE NUMBERS VARY, it appears that gestational diabetes affects 7 to 14 percent of all pregnant women. Official protocols in each state vary for the diagnosis and management of this disease and there is conflicting information about how to test, monitor, and treat gestational diabetes. The midwifery model of care demands individualized attention, which is why we push for testing, or other management practices, that exceed the standard practice. You and your midwife will decide together how to address these. The simple fact is that most gestational diabetes can be controlled by adjusting your diet and activity level—it is great that such a devastating disease can be avoided or corrected through a mother's own power!

What is diabetes?

DIABETES, WHICH IS SOMETIMES called diabetes mellitus, refers to a group of metabolic disorders. The word "diabetes" is derived from the Greek word meaning "to siphon, to pass through," and "mellitus" comes from the Latin word for "honey." "Mellitus" is often dropped and just the word "diabetes" is used when referring to the disease. Diabetes is a nutritional disorder characterized by an abnormally high level of blood glucose (blood sugar) and the excretion of the excess glucose in the urine. These high levels of blood glucose lead to difficulties with carbohydrate metabolism.

What is carbohydrate metabolism?

WHEN CARBOHYDRATES ARE METABOLIZED, the body breaks down the starches you eat and converts them to glucose (a simple sugar). Glucose is the primary nourishment for cells and is needed by the body for energy. Pancreatic cells regulate the use of glucose throughout the body by producing a hormone called insulin. Insulin functions as a gatekeeper, which allows or denies glucose access to the cells. When glucose does enter into the cells, it combines with oxygen to create carbon dioxide and water. This process releases energy, which is used for maintaining body temperature and taking care of nerve tissue (especially in the brain).

How does insulin work during pregnancy?

TO ENSURE THAT YOUR developing baby gets the nutrition he needs, your pregnant body changes how it metabolizes carbohydrates, fats, ketones, and proteins. Together, the placenta, the mother's hormones, and the body fat that pregnant women have all help suppress insulin. As your pregnancy progresses, your pancreas generates more insulin to compensate. This allows sugars to stay in your bloodstream for long periods of time, which keeps them available for your baby's growth and development. This process peaks in the last trimester, when your baby is putting on weight and needs support for all of that growth.

The placenta is thought to play an important role in regulating glucose delivery to your baby. All of these changes result in your glucose levels measuring the same or higher than a nonpregnant woman after a meal. Fasting glucose levels will also rise as pregnancy advances. *This is all normal and healthy.*

This finely tuned system will not work if your insulin-producing cells are damaged. Your pancreas will resist the entry of insulin (referred to as insulin resistance). The cells throughout your body begin to starve from lack of nourishment, which is why untreated diabetes leads to the failure of a variety of organs in the mother and multiple complications for the baby.

I had type 2 diabetes before pregnancy began; how will this affect me?

A MOTHER WITH TYPE 2 diabetes who can maintain normal fasting and postprandial (after a meal) blood sugar levels through diet and exercise has very little increased risks with her pregnancy. You should test more frequently as your body will change with the advance of pregnancy. At the 24th week, a postprandial lab test can confirm the home-test findings. Your midwife can help you to adjust your nutrition and exercise regimens. If you are unable to control your blood sugar levels without the use of insulin, you will fall into the same risk category of a woman with type 1 diabetes (see facing page).

I had type 1 diabetes before pregnancy began. How will this affect me?

TYPE 1 DIABETES CAN only be controlled through the use of the medication insulin. Blood sugar levels can change significantly quite quickly during pregnancy and labor, and careful control is required for your health and the health of your baby. It is very rare for a midwife to feel comfortable with a homebirth for a type 1 diabetic mother.[24]

> I had always dreamed of having my babies at home, so when I became pregnant I went to a homebirth midwife that had a great reputation in my community. During our first meeting she asked about my general health history. I told her I have type 1 diabetes. She explained the challenges with my condition and keeping my blood sugars steady through labor and delivery. She did not, however, just throw me to the wolves! She helped me find a great hospital-based midwife and a doula who understood homebirth and helped me create a great environment in my hospital room. We bought battery-powered "candles," took pictures of our dogs with us, and I wore my own beautiful nightgown instead of the standard hospital garb. It was a hospital birth but we did so well because of the guidance our homebirth midwife gave us!
>
> —Sadie

Can you define gestational diabetes?

GESTATIONAL DIABETES INCLUDES

- all diabetic diagnoses that are established after conception, either diet or insulin controlled
- transient impaired glucose regulation—sugar values in the range of true diabetes but that resolve after birth
- no longstanding diabetes damage to the maternal blood vessels or kidneys

Are there factors that increase the likelihood that I will develop gestational diabetes?

FACTORS THAT INCREASE YOUR risk for gestational diabetes are obesity, a family history of diabetes, having given birth to a very large infant previously, having had a stillbirth or a child with a birth defect, or having too much amniotic fluid. Women over twenty-five, those with a history of alcoholism, anorexia, bulimia, or nutritional deficits in their diet (or a diet based on white flour, white sugar, and processed food), and women who do not exercise regularly are also at increased risk.[25]

What are some symptoms of gestational diabetes?

- fatigue
- frequent urination
- excessive thirst
- blurry vision
- low blood volume
- ketoacidosis (an accumulation of ketones in the body)

What are the risks to the developing baby if gestational diabetes goes untreated?

DURING PREGNANCY, BABIES OF diabetic women can grow larger than others. When the mother's blood has too much glucose, the baby's pancreas produces more insulin in an attempt to use the glucose. The baby then converts the extra glucose to fat. The combination of high blood-glucose levels from the mother and high insulin levels in the baby results in large deposits of fat, causing the baby to grow quite large, especially in the face and shoulders. The biggest risks to babies of mothers with gestational diabetes are those associated with large babies: shoulder dystocias and cesarean birth—and all of the subsequent risks associated with surgical delivery.[26] Additionally, research has shown increased risk for premature rupture of membranes and breech positioning among diabetic women.[27]

Extremes of low and high blood sugar in early pregnancy can cause malformations or miscarriage. Undiagnosed, untreated gestational diabetes can lead to kidney complications, which can jeopardize the health of the fetus.

If the biggest risk is large babies, why don't all women with gestational diabetes just have cesarean births so they can avoid the danger to their babies?

THERE IS NO RESEARCH that supports the use of cesarean delivery to avoid birth trauma in women who have gestational diabetes. This is true for several reasons, but the most important one is the difficulty providers have in accurately knowing just how large a baby is before it is born. Ultrasound has a known error rate of 13 percent when it comes to estimating fetal weight.[28]

A provider who believes that your baby is 10 pounds could be off by as much as 1 pound, 3 ounces. While many providers might worry about a baby who they believe to be greater than 10 pounds, we would have to work really hard to find someone who believes a baby in the 8½- to 9-pound range is inherently risky to birth vaginally. The likelihood of a perfectly healthy vaginal delivery of this size baby is high.

Additionally, we cannot count the number of women we know personally who were told they needed a cesarean for an 11-pound baby only to birth an 8-pound child. There is significant grieving by women who make this decision trusting the ultrasound numbers and their provider, only to find themselves recovering from major abdominal surgery and longing for the birth they had planned.

Researchers looked at this issue and created a decision analysis that evaluated the cost and efficacy of a policy of elective cesarean delivery for an estimated fetal weight of 9 pounds, 15 ounces in mothers with diabetes. They found that 443 cesarean deliveries would need to be performed to prevent one case of birth injury caused by the baby's large size, at a cost of $930,000.[29] This shows that simply providing cesarean births for babies when a provider *thinks* they may be big does not result in safer births (and it costs much much more!).

What are the risks associated with gestational diabetes for the newborn?

DURING LABOR, HIGH BLOOD glucose in a mother with true and uncontrolled gestational or other diabetes will produce high insulin levels in the baby. This can cause his blood glucose levels to plummet immediately after delivery, since he no longer has the high sugar concentration from his mother's blood. If this goes uncorrected, midwife and textbook author Anne Frye says it can lead to "Tremors, respiratory distress, listlessness, abnormal crying, feeding difficulties, possible convulsions, and/or potential brain damage."[30] Babies of diabetic mothers can also be born with chemical imbalances such as low serum calcium or magnesium levels.

Babies who have been exposed to too much insulin (through an overuse of the treatment therapy in women who may not have actually needed it) can be born underweight and exhibit the symptoms of low blood sugar listed above.

What can a mother with gestational diabetes do to reduce the risks to her newborn?

THE BEST ANSWER IS early and frequent breastfeeding, which should balance out and prevent low blood sugar in your baby. A midwife should do a heel stick with a glucometer if she is at all concerned about your newborn's blood sugar levels. In the hospital, treatment for babies with low blood sugar ranges from a 12- to 24-hour NICU stay for the baby with heel pricks every half hour to three hours, until their levels return to normal.

Does gestational diabetes disappear after birth?

WHILE GESTATIONAL DIABETES TENDS to disappear after the pregnancy, it corresponds to a significant increase in the likelihood of adult-onset diabetes later in the mother's life.[31] Some studies report levels as high as 40 percent among women who had gestational diabetes going on to develop adult-onset diabetes. This may be due to the fact that many women with gestational diabetes fix in their minds that they have to make the diet and exercise changes only for the duration of their pregnancies; then, with relief that they "made it" through the end of the pregnancy, they return to pre-pregnancy lifestyle choices regarding nutrition and exercise. We encourage all expecting mothers, especially those with gestational diabetes, to approach the new way they handle diet and exercise regimes as a lifelong commitment that will potentially help avoid adult-onset diabetes.

A study published in 2011 revealed that new mothers who gained 12 to 17 pounds between their first and second pregnancies more than doubled their risk for gestational diabetes compared to women whose weight changed very little. Women who gained 18 pounds or more between births more than tripled their chances of developing this condition. On the other hand, losing weight before your next pregnancy may prevent gestational diabetes from recurring.[32]

Additionally, research has shown that gestational diabetes changes muscle physiology. Women with gestational diabetes who had cesarean sections have a significant increase in incontinence and decreased vaginal pressure two years post-cesarean, compared with women who were otherwise healthy but had cesarean births.[33] Diabetes alters the body in significant ways.

What kind of diet will give me the best chance of preventing gestational diabetes?

EACH WOMAN NEEDS TO work with her provider to establish the best diet for her specific needs. Generally speaking, to maintain steady blood sugars, one should eat small, frequent meals throughout the day. Each meal should have vegetables, fruits, and a lot of protein in addition to complex carbohydrates that are high in fiber. Salt a bit more than to taste, and drop simple sugars and carbohydrates from the diet. If you can, exercise some every day—preferably including short walks after every meal—it will help metabolize your food in a healthy way.

How should I test for gestational diabetes?

IN BOTH THE TRADITIONAL obstetric model and the midwifery model of prenatal care in America, all pregnant women are offered a screening for gestational diabetes. There are two types of tests typically offered. The first is the Glucose Challenge Test (GCT), which is actually a screen and not a test at all. To perform this screen, a woman is given a drink called Glucola, which has 50 grams of glucose in it, to drink the morning of her screen. She then arrives at the midwife's office or lab an hour later and has her blood drawn. If her blood sugar level is high, the woman will be asked to take the second test, the Oral Glucose Tolerance Test (OGTT).

The OGTT starts with a blood draw after an overnight fast of at least ten hours. The pregnant mother is then given 100 grams of glucose to drink and blood samples are taken after one, two, and three hours. If two or more values are high, the woman is considered to have gestational diabetes.

We do not have confidence in this test for many reasons, including the fact that it doesn't take into account the effects of a diet low in refined sugars, and several medications and medical conditions can influence the results. Its poor reproducibility has led the World Health Organization to state that this test should not be used for initial diagnoses of diabetes of any kind. This calls into question what kind of decisions you want to make based on such unreliable information.

I am a little embarrassed to admit this, but so many pregnant women do what I did, so at least I'm in good company! I have a great diet, low in sugars and simple carbs. I eat tons of veggies, chicken, and fish. I went in for my Glucose Challenge Test because the doctor told me to. I drank the drink they gave me in the lab. I thought I missed drinking soda in my life and was secretly looking forward to this drink. Surprise, surprise! Either my memory is really bad about what soda is like or this is just fourteen steps past disgusting. I knew right away it was going to be a problem. I was nauseated immediately and that feeling only intensified over the next hour. I had not had that much sugar of such low quality in my body since I had sugar cereal at sleepaway camp in the mid-'90s. It hit me like lightning. I could not stand up, and I felt sweaty and dizzy. They dragged me to the blood draw station and of course my levels came back high—my body had no experience processing that kind of sugar. I told them if they had me snort cocaine, I would probably react better!

I refused to do the OGTT—which was twice the amount that I had drunk for the first test. I felt really bullied by my doctor and to make a long story short, that was the final straw that sent me seeking midwifery care.

—Christine

Tests to Discuss with Your Midwife

FASTING GLUCOSE LEVEL. Research supports including a fasting glucose level at your initial appointment.[34] Repeating the test at 24 weeks and comparing it with this baseline level can provide valuable insight. These two tests show how your ability to absorb sugar has changed during the course of your pregnancy.

THYROID FUNCTION. Your thyroid should be tested. If it is working too fast or too slow, it can affect blood sugar regulation. This is a simple fact but the importance cannot be overstated. Undiagnosed thyroid conditions are prevalent among American women. Thyroid issues are one of the topics covered extensively later in this chapter.

URINE TESTS. Urine tests are important throughout pregnancy, which is why you will pee on a stick at every visit. The presence of both glucose and ketones early in pregnancy suggests diabetes that predates the pregnancy.[35]

As pregnancy advances, finding glucose in the urine becomes more common simply due to increased blood volume, which triggers the kidneys to release glucose at a lower threshold. Even so, if there is more than a trace, you should eliminate all refined sugars and test again two days later first thing in the morning. Then, don't drink anything, and test again two hours later.

POSTPRANDIAL TESTING. Assessing glucose levels after a normal meal is called a postprandial test and shows what is actually happening in your body on a typical day. This testing is done over the course of a week using a hand-held glucometer. The mother uses this small device to prick her finger one hour after each meal.[36] She can then enter her results into a diary to share with her midwife. She can also track which foods give great results.

HgA1c. Another test recommended in a lot of literature is the Hemoglobin (Hg) A1c test.[37] It should be given in combination with a fasting blood sugar test at the initial visit and again at the time of screening for gestational diabetes.

Bottom Line: How should I be tested for gestational diabetes?

ALTHOUGH THERE IS NO *evidence that supports being able to trust the results of the OGTT (oral glucose tolerance test), and this test offers far inferior information than the alternatives (see box opposite), it is the standard practice.*

If you or your midwife suspects trouble, the most effective testing is a combination of several tests. We suggest using the fasting blood sugar values from the initial visit and the 24-week visit, and the HgA1c in combination with a one-hour postprandial blood sugar test. Follow this with one week of testing at home an hour after meals. This plan will give you a complete and holistic picture of how your body is processing sugars.

As we discussed previously, blood glucose values rise naturally as pregnancy advances, but no adjustments are made for this in terms of the thresholds that result in a gestational diabetes diagnosis. Taking a test at week 28 might result in a failing level, while the same mother may have passed the test had she taken it in week 24. Take the test at the earliest time it is offered to get the most accurate results.

Wow. This seems like an enormous sinkhole and I do not want to fall in it. Are there natural options for avoiding or controlling gestational diabetes?

PREVENTING DIABETES THROUGH PROPER nutrition and regular exercise is the approach we recommend. Simply restricting calories is not the answer. Making sure that the calories you take in have a

> **The Midwife Says:** Midwifery expert Gloria Lemay says, "Whole organic foods, fresh water, and love are the ingredients to grow a healthy baby."

high nutritional value is.[38] Many practitioners (midwives included) tell women to "eat better and exercise more." This is not enough information. All of us need educational discussions, guidance, and help creating specific plans for meals and an exercise program.

A diet high in legumes (beans), nuts, and high-chromium food, such as broccoli, can help prevent gestational diabetes and control it once it has set in.

At my 16-week visit my midwife was worried about how I looked. I can't say I felt all that great, either. After some testing, it was clear that I had gestational diabetes. I absolutely freaked out. She told me that if I could not control it through diet and exercise that I would "risk out" of homebirth care. She was honest but kind about it. I felt guilty. I knew it must be bad for my baby. She helped me make a meal plan for the next two weeks. It included short walks after each meal, cutting out processed foods, sugar, and milk. She sent me home with a handheld finger-poker which measured how much sugar was in my blood. I had instructions to test before and after each meal and to record the results in a little diary she gave me.

At first I found it annoying to be poking myself all the time; just getting a grip on the new diet was a big challenge. But then I started to understand the numbers and how my activity level and food choices affected them. I have always been a bit of a rebel so I took delight when I felt I cracked the code to get low numbers. I stopped focusing on the hardship and started focusing on beating the machine! When I returned two weeks later, my midwife celebrated my success with me. She helped me find resources online so that I learned how to cook healthier and keep up what I had started. I tested myself one week out of every month for the rest of the pregnancy, never went back to those high blood sugar levels, and had the homebirth of my dreams!"

—Karen

Simple Foods for Healthy Blood Sugar

In addition to making a good meal and exercise plan with your midwife or nutritionist, you can make some simple additions to your intake every day:

- **MAKE STRING BEAN SKIN TEA.**
    - ★ *1 cup of tea made from the skin of string beans introduces inulin, a precursor to insulin, into the bloodstream. Jerusalem artichokes thinly peeled and sautéed provide the same nutrients.*

- **B$_6$ IT UP.**
    - ★ *A family history of diabetes can point to a genetic tendency for a woman's estrogen to bond to insulin if there is also a deficiency in vitamin B$_6$ (100-milligram doses of vitamin B$_6$ three times per day can uncouple the estrogen and allow the insulin to be used properly).*
    - ★ *It is estimated that vitamin B$_6$ plays a role in more than one hundred chemical reactions in our body, including helping releasing glucose from our cells.*
    - ★ *Vitamin B$_6$ creates amino acids, which build proteins, essential for the repair and growth of our tissue. It helps the body make serotonin, norepinephrine, dopamine, and GABA—all important neurotransmitters for pregnancy and birthing. Vitamin B$_6$ also helps with vas-*

cular health and metabolizing our food into
energy.

▲ Get your vitamin B$_6$ levels tested and make
a treatment plan with your midwife.

▲ Foods rich in vitamin B$_6$ include rice bran,
sesame seeds, chickpeas, wheat bran, bananas, salmon, avocado, dark turkey meat,
acorn squash, spinach, and raisins.

- **STEEP THE CINNAMON.**

  ★ Cinnamon has been shown to have hypogly-
  cemic (lowers blood sugar levels), antioxidant,
  and insulin-enhancing properties.[39]

  ★ It is safe to consume during pregnancy (even
  according to the conservative FDA).

  ▲ Make your own infusion by boiling cinnamon with water. Dried cinnamon should have
  2 teaspoons per 1 cup of boiling water. Cinnamon seeds should be brewed with 2 teaspoons of seeds per 1 cup of boiling water. If
  bark is used, 1 tablespoon per cup of boiling
  water. (Bark is what we commonly think of as
  a cinnamon stick. Grind for best results.)

- **ADD IN THE ONION.**

  ★ Onions have allicin and allyl propyl disulfide,
  which help block sudden increase in blood
  sugar levels.

  ▲ Work them into salads, veggie side dishes,
  and main courses throughout the day.

- **GET YOUR BROCCOLI ON.**

  ★ *Broccoli offers chromium, an essential mineral that facilitates the entry of glucose into the cells by working with insulin.*

  ★ *Broccoli is sometimes called a miracle food because it has the additional benefits of being iron rich; is high in vitamin C, folic acid, potassium, carotenoids; and is high in fiber.*

    ▲ *Eat it raw or steam it in the morning and munch all day long but keep it green— overcooking sucks out all of the nutrients.*

- **COUNT YOUR BEANS.**

  ★ *Beans are high in complex carbohydrates and fiber.*

  ★ *Black beans are the superstar of the bean family, packing in a high percentage of vitamins and minerals.*

  ★ *When combined with a whole grain such as brown rice, they form a perfect almost-fat-free meal.*

  ★ *Research has shown that some type 2 diabetics were able to stop using insulin just by getting more beans in their diet. In the same study, type 1 diabetics were able to reduce its use by 38 percent when they added beans to their diet.[40]*

  ★ *Black beans help prevent blood sugar from rising quickly after a meal.*

- **GET TO KNOW THE GLYCEMIC INDEX AS A GENERAL GUIDE.**
  - ★ *Good food choices are those that have low glycemic values, offer plenty of nutrients, and are lower in calories. Go to www.glycemicindex.com to see what the glycemic index is for your favorite foods.*

  - ★ *Foods that are ranked high on the index are followed by a quick and significant increase in blood sugar.*

  - ★ *Foods that are ranked low on the index will release glucose slowly and steadily into the bloodstream.*

    - ▲ *Quality and quantity both matter—get to know the right amount of the right foods to eat for your best health during pregnancy, nursing, and beyond.*

- **EXERCISE HELPS INCREASE GLUCOSE UPTAKE INTO THE CELLS OF MUSCLES REGARDLESS OF INSULIN LEVELS.**
  - ▲ *Head out for a ten-minute walk after each meal.*
  - ▲ *Add swimming or sustained walking into your weekly schedule.*

This is a lot of information. What is the take-home message?

IT IS CLEAR, FROM studies, common sense, and intuition, that there is one course to reduce any risks associated with high blood sugar to the mother and the baby: (1) make sure that the calories you ingest are nutrient dense and (2) exercise regularly. If you do any testing, use a combination of tests to give you a broad and holistic understanding of how your body processes sugar.

The Thyroid

A HEALTHY THYROID IS vital to the health of your body, your pregnancy, and your baby. This little butterfly-shaped organ, located just below your Adam's apple, regulates the energy used by your entire body and is in charge of your metabolism. The thyroid produces thyroid hormones and helps a variety of other hormones to do their work properly, and it requires iodine to function. Think of a car. A car with a full tank of gas but no gas pedal is just two couches and a roof with some nice storage room. Your body without great thyroid function lacks the vitality and efficiency it needs to keep you well, support a pregnancy, and grow a healthy baby.

While there are several variants of thyroid dysfunction and thyroid diseases, we will discuss the two basic types of impaired thyroid function that are most likely to crop up during pregnancy. The first is *hypo*thyroid (underactive) and the second is *hyper*thyroid (overactive) dysfunction. If you are diagnosed with thyroid problems, your physician will educate you as to the exact type of dysfunction, how it is caused, and the treatment for it.

There is not a consensus among midwives as to whether or not to offer thyroid tests during pregnancy. A study of more than 1,500 women showed that if *only* those pregnant women with personal or family history of thyroid diseases were tested, only 70 percent of women with hypothyroidism would be identified.[41] Ask your parents if there is a history of thyroid dysfunction in your family, and for whatever reason, if you do want testing, discuss the options with your midwife or provider.

What is hypothyroidism and how does it make you feel during pregnancy?

HYPOTHYROIDISM IS THE CONDITION that occurs when there is a deficiency of either the thyroid hormones known as TSH (thyroid-stimulating hormone) or TRH (thyrotropin-releasing hormone). The deficiency can range from so mild that a person can experience very subtle symptoms to quite severe, including multisystem organ failure. For most women, hypothyroidism presents as a feeling of sluggishness or fatigue, hair loss, abnormal weight gain, and intolerance to cold. Rough skin, difficulty with memory, decreased libido, and constipation are also common symptoms.

It can be hard to distinguish regular pregnancy concerns from a real thyroid problem. Some symptoms of pregnancy are quite similar to hypothyroidism: Pregnancy can make you feel very tired, skin changes often occur, and many moms experience memory issues. Constipation or other digestive issues can be normal during pregnancy, too. But your weight gain should be slow and steady, your hair should increase in luster and volume, and, if you are like most pregnant women, you will feel warmer than normal. When it comes to sex drive, many women report increased libido in the second trimester of pregnancy.

There is a class of this disorder called subclinical hypothyroidism that occurs when a person feels the symptoms of hypothyroidism but their blood work is all within normal limits. This is a known diagnosis and has been shown to create an increase in preterm delivery. If you have all of the symptoms but are told that you do not have hypothyroidism, it is important to follow up with a doctor, usually an endocrinologist, who understands and works with this particular condition.

Anytime you feel your body is responding to your normal daily activities in a way that doesn't make sense, make a note of it and share it with your midwife at your next prenatal visit. If you have symptoms that seem very abnormal, don't be shy about calling between visits. Your midwife would rather have you feeling safe and healthy by talking about your pregnancy than anxious and worried or missing out on the benefits of a good night's sleep.

What is hyperthyroidism and how does it make you feel during pregnancy?

HYPERTHYROIDISM IS THE OVERPRODUCTION of thyroid hormones. It can be felt as heart palpitations, increased appetite with unusual weight loss, easy bruising, excess sweating, diarrhea, muscle weakness, and sensitivity to heat.

As we said earlier, it can be hard to distinguish regular pregnancy concerns from a real thyroid problem. During pregnancy you may feel ravenous at times, or lose some weight with the initial morning sickness. If you think you are eating much more than normal but losing weight, bring this to the attention of your midwife. Having loose stools is a normal pregnancy symptom, as is feeling lousy in the heat, but if your bowel troubles are excessive or if you faint, let your provider know right away. Regular exercise should not make you feel extremely weak or fatigued. It should help keep your muscles strong and enhance your feelings of well-being.

Is there a way to treat impaired thyroid function?

YES. THERE ARE MEDICATIONS that regulate the thyroid quite effectively and have been shown to virtually eliminate the risks to you and your baby. This is one reason why testing your thyroid is prudent if you suspect that something is wrong. The treatment is effective and affordable, and there are several options for treatment plans. You can work with an endocrinologist or naturopathic physician to find the right medication while continuing to receive midwifery care for your pregnancy. Your midwife will consult with your physician to make sure that you are safe for a homebirth and that all of your lab results are recorded into your pregnancy chart. If you go into pregnancy with a previously diagnosed thyroid condition and are on medication, it will most likely need to be adjusted during pregnancy. Maintain regular visits with your endocrinologist or provider to keep your levels even.

What are the problems that can occur for me if my thyroid isn't functioning correctly?

A QUICK REVIEW OF the symptoms listed above shows that mothers with thyroid disorders in either direction can feel pretty miserable and even become quite dysfunctional. A mother who cannot eat well, exercise regularly, enjoy social interactions, or feel a sense of well-being may come to feel that her pregnancy is harming her.

Furthermore, because hyperemesis (the inability to keep down any food or drink and a loss of 5 percent of your body weight) is associated with hyperthyroid, mothers can suffer from dehydration and lack of nutrition, and the subsequent consequences. Feelings of despair and guilt in addition to the physical symptoms can add up and become overwhelming.

Thyroid disorders can take a toll on a woman's entire life and in fact are often mistaken for clinical depression. Because treatment is so effective both at reducing the symptoms and consequences for mothers and babies, if you suspect your thyroid is off, bring it to your midwife's attention.

What are the problems that can occur for my baby if my thyroid is not functioning correctly?

EFFECTS ON THE DEVELOPING baby depend on the type of thyroid dysfunction a mother has. They can range from early miscarriage and preterm births (from hypothyroidism) to neurological damage (from iodine deficiency). Research has shown that normal brain development depends on healthy levels of maternal thyroid hormones.[42]

Are there any thyroid issues to be aware of during the postpartum time?

- Newborns whose mothers have Graves' disease, a form of hypothyroidism, may need to be evaluated during the immediate and ongoing postpartum time to measure their thyroid function as they adjust to life outside of the mother's hormonal influences.

- Women with gestational diabetes have a significantly increased risk for postpartum thyroiditis (PPT) and should be screened at three and six months postpartum.

- Women who have PPT are at increased risk for hypothyroidism in the future.[43]

- Women with postpartum depression should be screened for PPT to rule it out, since the symptoms of PPT and depression mimic each other.

- If you have been taking thyroid medication during pregnancy for any reason, it will most likely need to be adjusted after pregnancy and your levels should be screened at three and six months.

What kind of nutritional intake will support my thyroid?

THE THYROID NEEDS IODINE to function properly. Iodine is a trace mineral and is required by the body for the synthesis of the thyroid hormones. It is found most commonly in the American diet in the salt we eat, if we purchase salt that has been iodized. However, we have on the whole been warned against the use of salt in our diet, which may be causing many people in the United States and the developed world to become deficient in iodine.

In Japan, where women (pregnant or not) regularly eat iodine-rich seaweed, the average daily intake of iodine is 12.5 milligrams. As a whole, their society has much lower rates of the many diseases linked to iodine deficiency than its American counterpart.

We also need enough iodine in our diet each day so that the thyroid can help regulate our metabolism. We do not have research to show just how much iodine is optimal for pregnant women. We can, however, follow the Japanese standard with its proven health benefits and at least increase our daily intake. The measly amounts provided by most American diets just aren't enough.

Nutritional sources of iodine other than iodized salt include

- seaweed (especially kombu seaweed, which can be sliced and added to soups or stir-fry)
- yogurt
- whole, boiled eggs
- mozzarella cheese
- iodine supplements as recommended by your provider

"I think I'm just plain getting sick. What can I do?"

SNIFFLES, COUGHS, AND FEVERS are one part of life that marches forward regardless of the fact that you are pregnant. Obviously, if you are ill, you will want to consult your midwife. She knows your health history and your lifestyle and can give you personalized advice, including when to see a physician. In general, it is a good idea to refrain from over-the-counter drugs during the first trimester. There just hasn't been a lot of good research on the effect of these drugs in pregnant women (it can be, shall we say, ethically problematic to do so), and it is impossible to say how much of a certain medication is safe during which week.

What happens if I get sick? Can I take anything?

DURING THE FIRST 12 weeks, your developing baby is highly sensitive to substances that you ingest, vitamin deficiencies, and imbalanced hormones. After 12 weeks of pregnancy, the major organ structures are in place, although they are still immature. And while we all know how to avoid illness (wash your hands often, eat a healthy diet, keep up with your vitamins, and avoid crowds), at some point, you may find yourself sick. This chart lists some over-the-counter medications that are generally considered low risk for occasional use. We have also included some drugs that you should *not* take. This list is not all inclusive; we've just named the most common complaints and remedies. Check with your midwife before taking any supplement or medication.

ISSUE	LOW RISK	NOT SAFE
Heartburn, gas, upset stomach	Tums, Rolaids, Mylanta, Maalox, Gas-X	Pepto-Bismol
Headache, fever, pain	Acetaminophen (Tylenol)	Ibuprofen, Aspirin
Cuts and scrapes	Polysporin	
Topical itching	Benadryl (oral or topical), Hydrocortisone	
Constipation	Metamucil, Citrucel, Colace	Laxatives
Yeast infections	Gyne-Lotrimin 3, Lotrimin AF, Mycelex-7, Femstat 3, Mycelex-3	
Insomnia	Benadryl, Unisom Sleepgels Maximum-Strength, Nytol, Sominex	

ISSUE	LOW RISK	NOT SAFE
Cough and cold symptoms	Robitussin DM, Vicks Cough Syrup, Halls basic cough drops, Sudafed, Actifed	Halls Plus (Multi-symptom)

For those who prefer a more natural approach, at least as the first line of defense, this table is for you. The same caveats apply. Please check with your provider before taking any of these remedies, as she knows you best.

ISSUE	LOW RISK	NOT SAFE
Heartburn, gas, upset stomach	Papaya or pineapple enzymes, apple cider vinegar, water, lying on left side, knee/chest position	Greater celandine (herb)
Headache, fever, pain	Warm compress, ice, massage, arnica gel	Tiger balm
Topical itching	Calendula oil, aloe vera, calamine lotion, baking soda paste	
Constipation	Flaxseeds, Smooth Move Tea	Aloe juice
Yeast infections	Plain yogurt (by mouth or applied directly to affected area), acidophilus capsules	Tea tree oil

ISSUE	LOW RISK	NOT SAFE
Insomnia	Warm milk, meditation, relaxation exercises, peanut butter, chamomile tea	
Cough and cold symptoms	Honey and lemon in hot water, eucalyptus steam, neti pot, chicken broth, potato peel broth, horseradish, warm salt water gargle	Licorice root

Hypertensive Disorders

I keep hearing about a terrible pregnancy disorder called eclampsia. What is this?

ECLAMPSIA IS THE BIG bad wolf of pregnancy—almost every pregnant woman hears about it and anxiously asks for an explanation of it. Eclampsia is one of many disorders that affect the flow of blood in your body. There are several of these hypertensive disorders that can be of concern during pregnancy.

If you are reading older books or articles, the terms "pregnancy-induced hypertension" or "toxemia" were used to describe what we now call eclampsia. As science advances, we understand in greater detail how different disorders develop and progress, and we now have several known subcategories of eclampsia.

Let's take a brief look at the different types of eclampsia:

CHRONIC HYPERTENSION: This occurs when your
blood pressure is greater than 140/90 before or during the

first 20 weeks of your pregnancy. There will not be any protein detectable in your urine and your blood pressure will remain elevated for at least 12 weeks postpartum.

GESTATIONAL HYPERTENSION: This is hypertension that starts after the twentieth week of pregnancy. Your blood pressure will measure higher than 140/90 on at least two occasions no less than six hours apart.[44] There will not be any detectable protein in your urine but you may have swelling of the face, hands, and feet. This hypertension resolves quickly after the birth and it is only when your blood pressure returns to normal that an official diagnosis of gestational hypertension can be made.

PREECLAMPSIA-ECLAMPSIA: This disease is one of many you will find in the medical dictionary with a confusing hyphenated name. It is classified thusly to illustrate that preeclampsia is a precursor to eclampsia. For simplicity's sake we will use the term "preeclampsia" from here forward. It is diagnosed on a range from mild to severe dependent upon the degree of blood pressure elevation, the amount of protein in your urine, and the level of involvement of the cardiovascular system, liver, kidneys, and brain. Your midwife will likely ask you to collect your urine for twenty-four hours so that definitive tests can be ordered. The only known cure for preeclampsia is the birth of your baby. Treatment typically consists of specialized care, often in a hospital.

PREECLAMPSIA SUPERIMPOSED ON CHRONIC HYPERTENSION: This occurs if you develop preeclampsia that doesn't resolve after the birth. This diagnosis is usually made three months postpartum if your symptoms do not improve and you need ongoing medication for chronic hypertension.

What symptoms will I have if I develop preeclampsia?

WHILE THERE IS NO one symptom that indicates you have pre-eclampsia, there is a constellation of three symptoms that will alert your midwife to order some tests and dig deeper. These symptoms are

- high blood pressure—over 140/90
- protein in your urine (as seen on the urine dip sticks you use at each visit)
- swelling in the face and hands or generalized swelling

Each of these symptoms alone can be caused by a variety of pregnancy and non-pregnancy related conditions. For example, one-third of pre-eclamptic women will never have swelling but swelling is seen in a large percentage of the general population of pregnant women without preeclampsia.[45]

There are other symptoms of preeclampsia that require an urgent response. If you experience any of these, your midwife may order tests and perhaps transfer your care to an obstetrician or a hospital for further evaluation. These symptoms are

- rapid weight gain
- abdominal pain
- severe headaches
- blurry vision
- changed reflexes (either reduced or hyper)
- reduced or no urine output
- excessive nausea and vomiting after the twentieth week of pregnancy
- seizures
- swelling of your lung tissue, which can cause a deep cough or difficulty breathing

What is the treatment for hypertension or preeclampsia?

TREATMENT OPTIONS VARY DEPENDING on your exact condition. A wide range of choices, from at-home blood pressure monitoring to blood pressure (antihypertensive) medications, are available. Your midwife will work with you and will consult a physician for care if your condition escalates.

Studies have shown that for *mild* hypertensive disorders, the best outcomes result from taking low-dose baby aspirin (see below) and calcium supplements and being more watchful than usual. Weekly lab tests and non-stress tests or other ultrasound tests are commonly used to watch the baby's health.[46]

Are there certain risk factors that would make me more likely to get one of these conditions?

YES. RISK FACTORS FOR preeclampsia include preeclampsia with a previous pregnancy, maternal age above forty, twins (or multiple gestation), chronic kidney disease or hypertension, a high body mass index, antiphospholipid syndrome, and gestational diabetes.[47]

Is there anything I can do to avoid getting a hypertensive disorder?

IF YOU HAVE ONE of the high-risk factors listed above, research has shown that taking low-dose (baby) aspirin, under the supervision of a physician, can prevent preeclampsia and its consequences for the baby.[48] After researchers reviewed a variety of treatment plans and their outcomes, this was the only one shown to be effective for both Mother and Baby.[49] Talk with your provider about the proper dosage and care plan.

Other options include proper nutritional intake and supplementation, especially with calcium. It is important to talk with your provider about the best diet and supplements for you—there are so many variables in taste preference, dietary restrictions, and other personal or medical considerations, that there is no single "best recommendation" for a specific diet or supplement regimen.

Can these disorders affect my baby?

YES. IF YOUR BLOOD flow is compromised, your placenta doesn't get the nourishment it needs to function correctly. It cannot provide the amount or quality of oxygen and nutrition your baby needs to thrive.

With hypertensive disorders, babies can be born prematurely or not develop properly. If you are moved to traditional obstetric care because this condition is severe, the physicians will weigh the risks of continuing with the pregnancy for you and your baby. If your baby is born before she is ready to maintain her heart rate, breathing, temperature, *and* nutritional needs on her own, she will stay in Intensive Care to receive support until she is able to. Typically, medications are given to the mother to keep her stable until at least 37 weeks so that the baby has time to mature.[50]

I don't have any risk factors but I want to keep my cardiovascular system healthy. What do you recommend?

EXERCISE AND A GREAT diet. After a while, it seems that during pregnancy this is the answer to most questions, and that's because it is! Commit to moving every day in a way that gets your heart pumping— a brisk walk or a swim seem to be the favorites among the mamas we know. Moms with older kids, especially toddlers, can struggle with finding the time for these activities. We encourage you to turn on your favorite dance music, set a timer for twenty minutes, and boogie with your kids. You'll work up a sweat and it's so much fun!

Work with your midwife to create an optimal diet. These basic preventative measures will leave you feeling great about all you are doing for yourself and your baby. It is never easy to stick with it, so build up good support at home and with girlfriends, and keep up the hard work!

Two universally great nutritional helpers for keeping blood pressures in check are cucumbers and cayenne pepper. The cucumber is full of nutrients such as potassium, magnesium, and fiber, as well as vitamins C, A, K, and folate. Start each day by cutting one into quarters, and eat it during the day as a snack. One per day with no dressing or oil on it seems to help keep the cardiovascular system perky.

Cayenne pepper is loaded with vitamins A, C, B complex, and the minerals calcium and potassium. It is so effective at equalizing the pressure in the cardiovascular system that it has been used to stop heart attacks and internal hemorrhaging. Besides keeping your blood pressure stable, cayenne is a great preventative measure against varicose veins and hemorrhoids, helps with digestion, and prevents migraine headaches—four very common complaints of pregnancy.[51]

The easiest way to ingest this hot pepper is to put ¼ to ½ teaspoon of cayenne pepper powder in 4 to 6 ounces of warm water with honey and lemon to taste, and drink. Once you start drinking, don't stop until it's all down. You can find a variety of cayenne pepper powders in the spice section at your local grocery store. Adjust the amount and heat of the powder until you find one that is right for you.

Are there other hypertensive disorders to be concerned about?

SOME RARE DISORDERS THAT are seen during pregnancy are life threatening and require immediate hospitalization for medical treatment. They include the following:

- HELLP SYNDROME is an offshoot of severe preeclampsia and includes these conditions: hemolysis, elevated liver enzymes, and low platelets (HELLP). It primarily affects women with very severe preeclampsia, less than 1 percent of all pregnancies.

- ACUTE FATTY LIVER OF PREGNANCY (AFLP) is extremely rare, develops in the third trimester, and includes vomiting and jaundice as symptoms.
- PERIPARTUM CARDIOMYOPATHY (PPCM) is rare but has a high mortality rate. PPCM is heart failure that occurs within the last five months of pregnancy. The causes are unknown but may result from a viral infection in the heart. Obstetricians and cardiologists work together to manage the care of women with this disorder.

Is a hypertensive disorder responsible for the new spider veins on my leg?

YES. MANY PREGNANT WOMEN develop spider or varicose veins during pregnancy that do or do not resolve after the birth. These are normal.

If the veins hurt, feel hot to the touch, or you notice that one leg is more swollen than the other, contact your midwife and tell her about these symptoms.

We like to think of spider and varicose veins, along with stretch marks and the freakish ability to carry your baby *and* twenty items in one hand, as gifts that our babies leave us with. So plan on getting a baby *and* a stretch mark (or two) and perhaps some spider or varicose veins from the next sibling.

Unless these changes cause you pain, they are badges of honor, ladies! Sit up straight and take notice: in many cultures around the world, these changes in the body signal success in a woman's life— these are signs of achievement and glory. Your body is designed to stretch and change. It does this to accommodate *life*. These small reminders provide a remembrance of very profound and meaningful work.

Miscarriage

I had an early miscarriage and felt such a big loss. Is this normal?

FIRST, WE ARE SORRY for your loss. The loss of an early pregnancy is common, but that doesn't make it easy. We understand that your heart was already connected to your baby. Hopes and dreams bloom with the first signs of pregnancy. It is normal to grieve after a miscarriage, regardless of how early or advanced the pregnancy was. It is good and honorable.

Grief can be difficult for both the mother and the father, as well as for any siblings that were aware of the pregnancy. It is also common to feel a surge of grief on related anniversaries—the estimated due date for the baby you lost, the anniversary of the discovery of the pregnancy, as well as the anniversary of the loss itself.

Discussing the loss with others will often help alleviate your grief. Schedule an appointment with your midwife to talk about your miscarriage. She can provide reassurance and be a sounding board for you and your husband or partner as you work through your grief. Other women find comfort in talking with friends and family, which often means telling them that you were pregnant and lost the baby in the same conversation. You can also find online support groups that will connect you with other women who have experienced loss.

Is there a reason why I miscarried?

WOMEN NATURALLY WANT TO understand why they had a miscarriage. Some are wracked with unnecessary guilt and blame themselves. It's hard enough to lose your child; don't put yourself through self-blame, too. Most losses are due to genetic or developmental anomalies early in pregnancy, and there is nothing you could have done to change the outcome.

Note: While the cause is often unknowable, evaluation of the tissue for chromosomal anomalies is possible, although not the norm.

I had an early miscarriage and feel just fine emotionally. Does this mean I will be a bad mother to my future children or that I didn't love this baby?

THERE IS ABSOLUTELY NO right or wrong way to feel after a loss. If you feel grounded and stable, you are. There is no reason to believe you will be anything but a wonderful parent when the time comes.

I have had two miscarriages. Am I at a higher risk to miscarry again?

NO. YOUR RISK DOES not increase until you have had three miscarriages in a row. That said, there is no harm in having a complete workup to check your hormone levels and overall health. Women tend to feel better about their fertility if they know they are in good health and primed for pregnancy. Additionally, a post-miscarriage, preconception visit will allow you to ask any lingering questions, learn about risk factors, and address any ongoing health problems that may affect future pregnancies. We recommend naturopathic physicians or family practice doctors because of their tendency toward comprehensive, holistic, and positive perspectives when it comes to finding balance and well-being.

I had a miscarriage last month. Do I need to wait for a certain period of time before trying to conceive again?

THERE IS NO APPLICABLE evidence to indicate that there is any increased risk in getting pregnant again right after miscarriage. A small study conducted in 2002 looked at sixty-four pregnancies after miscarriage and found no evidence of pregnancy complications in those who conceived immediately compared to those who waited two cycles.[52] Additionally, a 2003 study found evidence that women might have increased fertility in the cycle immediately after a miscarriage.[53]

Providers often recommend waiting one to three months before trying for a new pregnancy: the main reason for waiting is your emotional health. If you feel strong emotionally and are in good health, then there is no medical reason to postpone trying again. Ask yourself: Do you feel ready? Does your partner? We recommend that all women take 400 micrograms of folic acid before trying to conceive, and 600 to 1000 micrograms once pregnant.

> I'm so blessed to have been under midwifery care when I experienced both my miscarriages. The love and support she (and her backup midwife) gave me was amazing . . . and essential! I know of no other provider who would sit on the phone with me crying (multiple times) as I experienced the contractions and was losing my babies. She checked up on me for weeks after, and was a huge source of comfort for me.
>
> —Carla

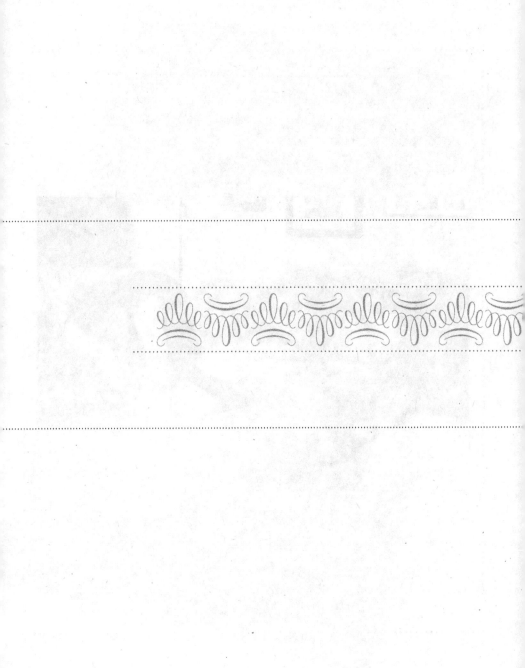

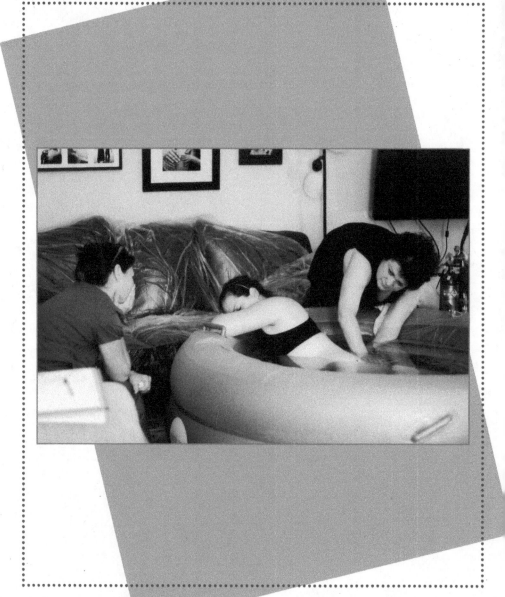

CHAPTER TEN

Labor and Birth at Home

- Preparing your home for the birth
- Birth kits
- Siblings at the birth or no siblings at the birth? That is the question!
- After the due date
- Labor and birth

MAMA SAYS

Homebirth is the absolute best decision I have ever made for my family. It brought us all together in ways that still resonate years later. It was so intense yet so gentle, which, not coincidently, I'm sure, is exactly who I am as a mother.

—Evangeline

Preparing Your Home for the Birth

PREPARING FOR AND HAVING your homebirth should be exciting, magical, challenging, and rewarding work. In this chapter we help you with specific tasks for nesting and preparing your home, children, and pets for the big day. We discuss early labor signs and offer some suggestions for how to care for yourself during this time. We share our tricks of the trade for laboring, waterbirth, and managing a transfer to the hospital should it be needed.

Exactly how do I prepare our home for my homebirth?

DON'T HATE US, BUT your mother-in-law is right to run her finger along your windowsill. Dusty windowsills do not mean you will be a horrible mother, but there really is something to having a clean home when you are planning to birth there. Midwives vary in just how strict they are, and in the methods they use to ascertain how clean your home is on a typical day. Some never ask about it and just deal with whatever they find when they arrive for the birth. On the other end of the spectrum, some may ask to come for an in-home prenatal visit just to get a sneak peek at your cleanliness.

When your midwife asks you about the state of your home (or anything else) during your prenatal visits, be honest with her. Her goal is your best health, and she is a great resource to help you make changes in your life. Follow the checklist below to succeed in prepping your homebirth home. Before you worry about how you'll get it done, remember that expecting mothers tend to have spouses, partners, or support people who are itching for ways to help. Say "Yes!" to them! And if that fails, you can count on the nesting instinct that kicks in a week or so before labor starts. Most baby-in-the-belly mamas are shocked by this sudden burst of energy and the desire to clean in the following ways:

- Declutter.

  + *Piles of mail, stacks of papers, books with nowhere to go? If it doesn't have a place and a purpose, get cold-hearted, get over it, and get it gone.*

- Dust first.

  + *For a few dollars you can purchase the handy and effective little Swiffer Dusters at your local grocery store. Start at the high points and dust down—wait, what are we saying? Hand the box of dusters to your partner or hubby, grab a girlfriend, and go to a movie. Be sure to tell him to start at the high points and hit every horizontal surface between the ceiling and floor.*

- Clean the floors, please.

  + *Midwives will spend the bulk of their time in your home on your floors. Couches are cushy and sofas are swell, but most mothers labor in such a way that it is more conducive to sit on the floor. No one likes to have to wipe dust, dirt, and dog hair off of their rear end when they stand up.*

- Scrub the potty.

  + *Cleaning the bathrooms is just the right thing to do. And by the way, if you aren't crazy about all the fumes from store-bought brands, just dilute white vinegar into water for all of your cleaning needs. Hit the toilets with a brush and cleaner, wipe the mirrors, wash the tubs, scrub the sinks, and mop the floors. At some point during your labor, you will be sitting on the toilet with your midwives and doula in the bathroom, too, as you work through some contractions there. Laboring on the toilet is a trick of the trade. A laboring mother who sits on the toilet tends to make oodles of changes to her cervix and the baby's position. You really want your midwife to be looking at you and not to be thinking about balancing on her heels so that she doesn't rest her hands on any half-dried man pee.*

- Tidy the kitchen.

  + *Wipe the counters, the stove fan, and the sink. Put away the dishes and clear the trash and the compost bins in early labor. Your midwife or doula will be in that kitchen fixing you up some tasty treats to nibble on throughout labor—prep it for them by getting it all clean.*

- Keep the mystery alive.

  + *Put away very personal items. There will potentially be quite a few people in and out of your room and pictures taken there on the day you have a baby. If these are things you don't care if you share with everyone, by all means let your freak flag fly—we can handle it. We may giggle about it later among ourselves, but it will come from a place of love.*

- Layer the bedding.

  + *In early labor, consider the fantastically distracting activity of making the bed. You likely will not birth your baby on your bed. You'll probably be on your hands and knees leaning forward onto the sofa, in the tub, or in a standing squat in your favorite room in the house. But you will want to get into your bed after the action is through, and it's always good to plan for every contingency. So here are the layers to place on your bed— stick with the order, it really works:*

    ❖ *mattress cover*

    ❖ *bottom sheet*

    ❖ *top sheet*

    ❖ *shower curtain or tarp*

    ❖ *bottom sheet*

❖ *top sheet*

❖ *light blanket folded down to the end of the bed*

✦ *After you are all cleaned up and ready to cuddle and get cozy as a family, your team will peel off the top layer of grubby sheets and the shower curtain. So cozy!*

What should I pack in case we need to transfer to the hospital?

IF YOU TRANSFER TO the hospital, you will want the following items on hand:

- warm socks
- a comfy pillow, a pillowcase that is not white to avoid hospital linen confusion
- a picture or two of the people or pets you love
- a hospital-based birth plan
- clothing and food for yourself and Dad
- clothing for the baby
- car seat for the baby

What should we do with the dog during our homebirth?

LET YOUR MIDWIFE KNOW ahead of time that you have a dog or any pet. Some are allergic and need to bring their allergy medicine. If your pooch growls, barks, or bites guests, it is best they are away from the birthing mother and her attendants. If your dog is stinky or annoying to you, park that puppy in another room, at the neighbors, or at the kennel. If you anticipate enjoyment of sharing the experience with your dog, there's a pretty good chance that you are in for some special moments.

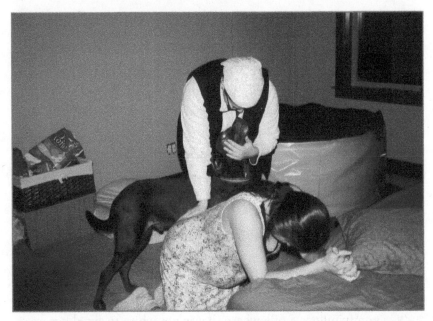

A classic pooch move: nosing in to help out with comfort measures.
Jodilyn, mom Tiffany, and dog Cape work through labor together.

The family dog can often work quite effectively at calming Mom—she can pet or even lean on the dog during contractions. After all, in many cases, the dog was the first baby in the family!

And what about the cat?

CATS, UNLIKE THEIR CANINE counterparts, seem to stay out of the way. They dart through the birth scene and give us a fright, leap off of counters, or stare at us suspiciously before retreating to wherever cats really go. Jane once saw a distressed cat jump across the stove and light itself on fire on the gas burner, but we are pretty sure that is not the norm. Like any pet, the solution can be found in your knowledge of their disposition, their ability to take a hint, and potential places to park the animal during labor if the mom wishes it to be out of sight.

Should we have anything at the house for our birth team during labor?

IT'S IN YOUR BEST interest to keep your midwives fueled. Ask your midwife what her expectations are. The answer may range from a ten-course meal to nothing but running water. Here are some unspoken truths about this issue: At the very moment you call your midwife to say you are in labor, she is either sitting down to eat, stepping into the shower, or finally going to bed after a twelve-hour workday. Having something to keep us going is always appreciated. Our favorite choices are lots of veggies and fruits, and healthy options that have a high nutrient value for each calorie ingested. While you are working through labor, we are preparing for the moments you will need us most—right at birth and during the immediate postpartum period. The last thing we need is doughnuts or pizza, which make us feel sluggish and nauseated at three in the morning. However, a side dish with some dark chocolate on it never seems to go untouched.

> **The Midwife Says:** Setting out a good spread is a great assignment for grandparents, and gives them a chance to ask the midwifery team questions and share their birth stories.

Birth Kits

We've read about "birth kits." What should we have in ours?

EVERY MIDWIFE WILL HAVE her own list of what to put into the birth kit. A birth kit is a group of items that your midwife deems necessary for homebirth. It can be put into a box or bag made from cardboard, paper, or plastic, and may require more than one container. A birth kit can be assembled by gathering bits and pieces from your local grocery store and pharmacy or by ordering supplies online. Some midwives sell birth kits that contain all of the supplies they prefer to have on hand. Others have a relationship with online retailers that you can purchase from.

Meanwhile, here are some common components of most birth kits:

- COLD AND HOT PACKS: These feel good in a variety of ways at a variety of times throughout the birth.

- ELECTROLYTE GEL: Cyclists, marathon runners, and hikers all use this Jell-o-like substance, which is essentially a concentrated electrolyte drink. It goes down easily and works quickly.

- FLEXIBLE STRAWS: For most laboring women, it is easier to drink from a straw than a cup.

- SHOWER CURTAIN: This goes onto the bed as explained previously.

- A FULL-SIZE, CLEAN, STURDY COOKIE SHEET OR CUTTING BOARD: It provides a firm surface for resuscitation if needed.

- AN ELECTRIC HEATING PAD: This is used to keep baby blankets warm and ready for after the birth. If necessary, it will also be placed on the surface used for resuscitation to keep the baby warm. This is why you may see a cookie sheet stacked with layers of blankets, heating pads, and then more blankets.

- LARGE SANITARY PADS: Used by the mom after the birth.

- LARGE, SOAKED AND FROZEN SANITARY PADS: Take a few cheap pads and unfold them on a cookie sheet. Drench them in witch hazel and place the cookie sheet in the freezer. When the pads are frozen, you can fold them up and put them into a plastic bag in the freezer. This soothing pad will make you say "Aaaahhhhh!" after birthing.

- INCONTINENCE UNDERGARMENTS: Adult diapers are really helpful for the first few days after birth because you don't have to wash them if there is some overflow from the sanitary pad. Place the pad in them and pull them on like regular underwear.

- BABY THERMOMETER: A baby's temperature is a window into his health. A low or high temp can tell Mom and Dad to use more or less clothing or can be indicators of infections in a newborn. A normal reading can provide you with a lot of comfort and reassurance about your healthy baby.

- UNDERPADS (ALSO CALLED CHUX PADS): These large blue, green, or white pads are found in the incontinence section of your local pharmacy. Put them underneath you to protect your bedding, sofa, and so forth. They keep everything clean and tidy and easily roll up for disposal.

- "PERI" IRRIGATION BOTTLE: This little squeeze bottle of yum will be your best friend. It is used to squirt warm water over your perineum while you pee in the postpartum time. It feels good and is the right thing to do for your body.

- FOUR DRAWSTRING KITCHEN GARBAGE BAGS: We typically use one for laundry and one for garbage, but we like extras to avoid rummaging if we need more.

- TOWELS: There are never enough of any-size towel at births. They are used throughout the birth and postpartum time—for drying off moms when they get out of the tub, lining the floor if Mom's water has broken, and stacking up for the midwife to sit on if she needs a break from a hard floor. Hand towels are used immediately postpartum to cover Baby as she is nestled in your arms. Washcloths can be soaked in ice water or hot water and draped over your forehead during labor for comfort. So have lots of bath-, hand-, and washcloth-sized towels on hand.

- BABY BLANKETS: For your baby!

The next two items on the list seem harmless enough but carry some controversy. Therefore, we want to examine some information regarding bulb syringes and baby hats:

- BULB SYRINGE: Some midwives never use these, and that is an intentional denial of a common practice. The physiological reality is that birth and babies are designed to work without the use of any outside suction sources. Babies are designed to clear their own airways and, in fact, need to. Their chests get a good squeeze in their final moments inside of you, which pushes fluid from their lungs and starts the breathing process. The sputters, coughs, and cries they give are designed to push open their lungs. They transition your baby from a fluid-filled environment to one where they are required to breathe air. Research has shown that the use of bulb syringes or any suction (even in the hospital) does not improve outcomes.[1]

  The first oral stimulation a baby receives should be his mother's breast (or sucking his own hand) and generally it's best to not overstimulate him right after birth. It is a huge adjustment for a baby to come from the soft, contained experience in utero into the bright, loud, rough-surfaced world we live in. Babies deserve to make that transition in the soft arms of their mothers, without plastic bulbs up their noses or in their mouths. Your midwife should carry her own suctioning equipment in case she feels the need to use it as a resuscitative measure. Ask her what her normal protocols are.

- BABY HAT: Oh, the baby hat! It's little and cute, and
  moms pick them out in all sorts of colors and patterns. But
  sometimes these little cuties can interfere with the most
  natural of processes; newborn babies and newly minted
  mothers are so interdependent upon each other that we
  think of them as one being: mother/baby. Immediately
  after the birth, we swoop the baby up to his mother's chest
  where he has his best shot at regulating his temperature,
  heart, and respiratory rates.[2] Some critical and thrilling
  events are happening in that moment.

Authors Marshall and Phyllis Klaus point out that, "All sorts of exchanges between the mother and infant are going on. The baby is taking in the mother through many senses, as is the mother learning about her baby. The baby is becoming familiar with the mother's smell and within a few days will pick out his or her mother's breast pad from other women's breast pads. This is related to the particular smell of one's own mother, not her milk."[3]

Incredibly, within the first day of birth a mother can pick out her baby by smell. These powerful olfactory workings are finely tuned to bond mother to baby, and baby to mother.[4]

We don't like to interfere with that process. If a mother is having a particularly tough time with coming back into her head after the birth, we will encourage her to lean down and take a big sniff of baby. Invariably, this wakes her to her baby and sets her on the course of cooing and admiring that every new mom and baby is entitled to experience. A hat can interfere with this crucial time.

I'm so green you might think Kermit is my first cousin. Is there anything I can do to have my homebirth "go green"?

THE TRICK WITH GOING green is to replace disposables with washables. If this is your choice, have extra laundry bags or baskets on hand and let your midwife know your plan. That said, here are some simple ideas for keeping your birth down with Mother Earth:

- Use laundry hampers or baskets instead of garbage bags for dirty linens.

- Purchase your extra towels and sheets at a consignment shop: adding half of a bottle of hydrogen peroxide to each load of laundry *with* your soap will almost always remove any staining, so that you can donate them back when you are done.

- Purchase fabric chux pads and sanitary napkins: you can find these online at etsy.com by searching for "underpads" and "sanitary napkins." You can wash and reuse these for years.

- Rent a birth tub from your midwife or a local rental company instead of purchasing your own: new liners are used for each mother so you will have a perfectly sanitary tub and create less waste in the process.

- There are lots of friendly household products to maintain a green home; if that's what you have in your home, that's what we'll use for your birth.

Siblings at the birth or no siblings at the birth? That is the question!

THIS IS SOMETHING THAT most families ponder when expecting a new baby. There are a lot of pros and cons, and the right answer depends on your family's communication and belief system. We can tell you that siblings at births seem to do best when:

- they feel safe and welcome to come and go as they'd like to
- they have a provider there just for them with whom they have a good relationship
- they have been told ahead of time things they can say and do to make Mama feel good and have practiced those phrases (Just learning to say, "Good job, Mama!" is a great task for a toddler, while offering cold washcloths is something older kids can do that provides meaningful comfort for Mom.)
- they have been exposed ahead of time to some of the loud noises Mom might make during labor (they can practice breathing and moaning with mom) and understand that these are good and normal noises. (Watching birth videos online together is a great way to accomplish this.)
- they have read books designed for siblings who are planning to attend a homebirth (See Appendix B for a list of current books on the market.)
- they have been given the language to talk about birth (These kids tend to know their anatomy and biology, and the science helps defuse the mystery and fear surrounding Mom's body.)
- they have been given the opportunity to attend prenatal appointments and participate in them by asking questions, helping the midwife measure Mom's belly, or listening to the baby's heart rate through the stethoscope

So what could possibly go wrong? If a child is distressed at the work of labor, or if she was well prepared but changes her mind and no provider is present, it can be very difficult for Mom. When this happens, the usual result is that Dad takes the sibling to another part of the house and the midwives and doula remain with the mother.

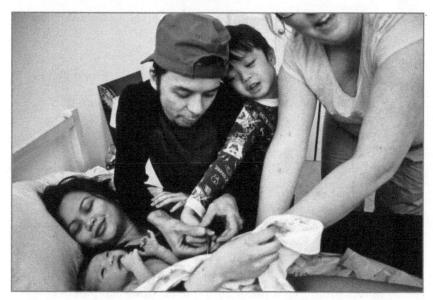

Daddy helps a well-supported and prepared Big Brother cut the cord.

Having a sitter at the birth ensures that you will get to share the birth with your partner.

At the birth of a fifth child on a typically rainy Seattle day, the older four siblings were all present. Their reactions to Mom in labor varied from excitement to total disinterest and shifted from moment to moment for each child. Mom and Dad had lots of support there for the kids in the form of aunts and uncles and grandparents.

The youngest sat with us for the whole labor, diligently watching her mother and holding our equipment for us. The next youngest was hardly in the room at all. The second to oldest and oldest alternated between time with Grandma and going over to check in on Mom. They knew ahead of time where to go to get close to her and what to expect from her.

When Baby was born, all of the siblings were present. The oldest daughter cried quite a lot. After Mom was settled in with Baby for the night, I asked the oldest daughter where her tears came from—happy, worried, relieved, etc. The girl replied, "I was so happy to see my mama bring me a baby sister. She worked so

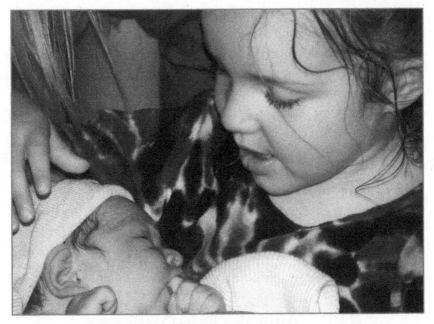

The Big Sister gets a thorough look at her new baby.

hard and she did good. I'm relieved she did it." This was a pretty sophisticated expression of fear, triumph, and empathy. It was born of that family's openness to sharing the heart, science, and details of homebirth well in advance of the big day.

The kids wanted to inspect the placenta, so I held a Placenta 101 workshop in the kitchen for them. Several of the aunts and the grandparents joined in. It was a great intergenerational learning experience and bonding time for all of them within the context of family and homebirth. It also gave Mom and Dad some quiet time with their newest baby.

—Connie (midwife)

The house is clean, the dog is happy, and I have all of my supplies. Is there anything else to consider?

DEFINITELY! YOU! YOUR EMOTIONAL well-being is the final element needed for a healthy homebirth. Don't get us wrong—you don't have to be the picture of psychological perfection. Pregnancy and birth is a great time to work through issues that have come forward from your childhood or difficult experiences you have had in your life. There is something about the dividing of cells within that propels women to think about how they can let go of the harm done in the past or at least park it in a safe and healthy way.

We have seen a couple of methods that really work to address these issues. The first is to journal nightly. Telling your story creates health and healing, even if no one else reads it. The second is to read the book *Parenting from the Inside Out* by Dan Siegel and Mary Hartzell and to do the exercises offered at the end of each chapter. It is not easy work preparing to be a parent, but the thoughtfulness and discussions you will have while reading this book will pay off exponentially.

After the Due Date

I am overdue by a few days and my midwife is telling me I am about to risk out of homebirth. Why won't I go into labor?

AH, THE CRY OF the 42-week mama. We've all heard the stories of overdue women who went to the massage therapist, chiropractor, palm reader or dog groomer, ate spicy food or pineapple, had tons of sex, walked for miles, and immediately went into labor. Sounds great, right? Well, far be it from us to disparage anyone's experience, but please understand that nothing will put a mother into the kind of labor that results in vaginal birth if she is not already ripe and ready to go. This is due to a naturally occurring phenomenon called the oxytocin receptor system. This is the mechanism by which our body reads and agrees to use oxytocin to regulate our birthing process. Research has shown that our receptor sites work effectively enough only to create the kind of labor needed for a vaginal birth when we are actually just about in labor.[5] This is one of the many reasons that *simply waiting* may be the best alternative treatment plan.

Can I use alternative modalities to induce labor before my time runs out with my midwife?

ALTERNATIVE MODALITIES NEED TO be seen for what they are: a wonderful investment in your health, both physical and mental. Use of any of the natural induction methods should be seen as supportive of your body and baby, and not something that will override what you two are already doing so successfully. There may be something that helps your labor start—it might be the treatment or the way you relax from the treatment, or the time it takes to be seen from the time you book the appointment for the treatment. It can be difficult to reconcile trust in your body and your baby while trying every trick in the book to spur them into action. However, this framework of trust can help keep the environment of your body and your home the low-stress zone that is so fundamental to birthing.

If you find yourself frazzled from the waiting, sit quietly and tell yourself and your baby how you are feeling. Reassure Baby that you are ready and send her loving thoughts. Your strong baby within and your strong mama-self have carried you both to this point beautifully. Pharmaceutical induction agents should be used only after evaluating the likelihood that they will succeed using a tool known as the Bishop's Score. Your midwife can help you navigate these decisions.

Bishop's Score

THE BISHOP'S SCORE IS a simple grid used to evaluate the likelihood of an induction leading to a spontaneous, vaginal birth. Practitioners across the spectrum of obstetrics and midwifery rely on this effective and proven tool. It gives scores to various elements that have been shown to be favorable to labor and birthing. Favorable scores are considered those between 6 and 13, with many sources citing 8 or even 9 as the bottom line for when a woman should consider induction an option. Scores less than 5 are considered unfavorable for inducing, and hospital-based care will rely upon a cervical ripening agent to try to boost the score before other induction agents are used.

Your midwife will create a care plan with you heading into the final weeks or days of your pregnancy. If you are high risk, your provider will add an additional category to the chart below to compensate for your condition.

BISHOP'S SCORE	0	1	2	3
Dilation	Closed	1–2cm	3–4cm	5+cm
Length of cervix	>4cm	3–4cm	1–2cm	0cm
Consistency of cervix	Firm	Medium	Soft	—
Position of cervix	Posterior	Midline	Anterior	—
Station of baby's head in the pelvis	–3	–2	–1, 0	+1, +2

Labor and Birth

Okay! Now I'm completely ready. What are some signs that I'm in early labor?

FIRST-TIME MOMS IN PARTICULAR need some reassurance that they are not going to miss their labor. After all, things are happening *down there* almost all the time during the last weeks of your pregnancy. But really, with extremely rare exception, you will know. Even moms who have two-hour labors know when something has shifted inside them and birth is on its way. Loose stools and decreased appetite are signs that labor is close. Some women feel restless when their birthing time is near. You may fixate on finishing your last bit of nesting or feel the sudden and overwhelming need to talk with your girlfriends and your mother. You may want to sit in a dark quiet place in your home and do some yoga. One thing we can absolutely reassure you about: you will not miss your birth. Your body will eventually demand your attention and participation. However your labor starts, follow your body

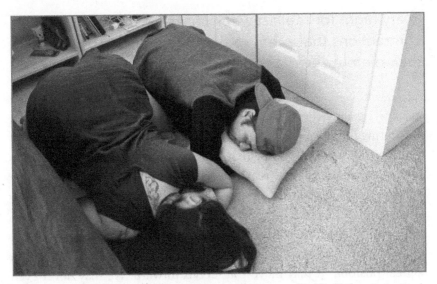

Mom and Dad take a break between contractions. Half of labor is resting!

where it takes you. It won't be long until you are holding your baby in your arms.

My belly tightens a lot. How will I know when it is really labor causing it?

YOU MAY HAVE BEEN having painless tightening for weeks. These squeezes are called Braxton Hicks, or, as we prefer to phrase it, warm-up contractions. They tone your uterus and give it a little bit of a workout before the big day.

Labor contractions are much more serious. They will get longer, stronger, and closer together as time passes. Labor is like a symphony. Put on some Beethoven or Mozart and you will notice a few elements that you can also expect during labor. Once it begins, it will increase in intensity and strength, crescendo, and then come to a calm and stunning finale. Just like the symphony doesn't stop or waver once it has begun, neither will your labor, although you may experience pauses between the movements. Warm-up contractions come and go. Labor that results in the birth of your child will not.

Every night for the last week I have been getting contractions that seem to get longer and stronger but then die out several hours later. I'm exhausted!

OCCASIONALLY MOTHERS MAY GET bouts of contractions that just don't go anywhere. This happens mainly at night, and can be very frustrating for all concerned. These contractions are known as prodromal labor or false labor, but that is rather insulting. There is *nothing* false about them. They're real, they hurt, and after several nights, they can really get on your last nerve. It can be helpful to know that every single contraction you have, whether it comes two weeks before your baby's birth or as the head slides out, is valuable and has a purpose.

Each contraction is doing something. It may move your baby into a great position. It may move your cervix forward. We may never even know what it is doing, and that is okay, too. But know that you are not contracting in vain. Every pain has a function. If you are experiencing repeat performances night after night, it may be that your baby is a little sideways or backward facing. You can help her straighten out by moving in ways that shift the diameter of your pelvis and her position in it. Spend time during the day on your hands and knees doing cat-cow yoga positions, resting with your rear in the air and your head on your folded arms, doing pelvic tilts and rocks, and swimming. To gain a great understanding of your pelvis, and your baby's position within it, we love the pelvic map work taught in The Pink Kit, found online at www.birthingbetter.com.

I had four nights of no-sleep, false-alarm contractions. I thought I would lose my mind. My husband had to work, which left me responsible for our two-year-old daughter. On the fifth day, I called my midwife for help. First of all, I learned that I should have called her after the first or second night, before my fatigue got so out of hand. She was so kind, even though I sort of sounded like a raving lunatic.

She assured me that all people sound that way after missing out on that much sleep. She helped me make a plan, which looking back, was so simple I should have thought of it. But when you are in the moment and that tired, it is hard to think clearly. I called in a babysitter and slept for the entire day. I woke up, made a hot and nutritious dinner with my husband, and then we put our daughter to bed, turned off the phones, and cuddled up and watched a movie.

When the contractions began again that night, I stuck my rear end in the air and rested in that position. I felt the baby move around a *lot* and after about a half hour the contractions died out and I fell back to sleep. I didn't go into labor for another four days, but something had shifted and I slept through the night (with the exception of emptying my full bladder) until then.

—Francesca

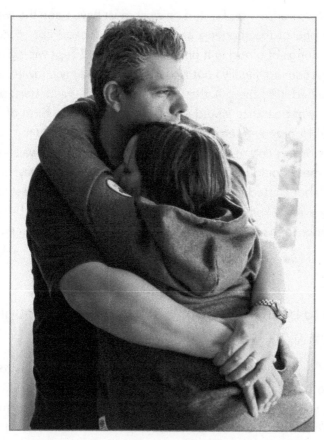

Mom leans in for some loving and support through a contraction.

There is bloody slimy goop coming out of my vagina. Am I going to have my baby now?

THE GOOD NEWS IS that you are getting closer to the time when she will make her appearance. You have officially lost your mucous plug, which serves to protect the uterus and baby from harmful germs for the duration of pregnancy. As your cervix begins to open, this plug begins to ooze out. The word "plug" is a misnomer—it is neither one piece nor something that drops out all at once, usually. It is a slimy, stringy, blood-tinged mucous that makes its appearance a few weeks, days, or hours before birth. Some women don't lose it until they are in active labor.

> What a surprise after I wiped on what must have been the twentieth pee of the morning and I saw what looked like mucous with strings of blood in it on the toilet paper. I kept wiping and it kept coming. Finally I put a pad in and called my midwife. She explained it as the gift that keeps on giving—what started as a slimy appearance would eventually end with the birth of our baby! Hooray, we were on our way! I loved seeing that my body was working and at the same time settled in for the wait—she told me it could be a week or two still. It was three days later that labor started and we had our homebirth (of the cutest little baby ever!). I know when I think of my birth, I will remember the confidence that first sign gave me that my body would work.
>
> —Katy

I seem to be in early labor, but it is not bad enough to stop me in my tracks. What should I do?

THE BEST THING TO do in early labor if it is daytime, is to ignore it and go have some fun! It's okay to stay home from work and give yourself some me-time. When we hear this question from mothers, we enthusiastically encourage them to go out to a movie—it will be a while before you can do that again. If not, watch a movie at home, take a walk, or go to the mall. Get your nails done! Do fun things with your partner, so you can look back happily on this time. Many couples make a nice meal and play a favorite board game. If you can rest or sleep, then do. Cuddle with your partner or take a warm bath together. Enjoy some last quiet moments of intimacy before your family changes. You will need a lot of energy in the coming hours. Use this time to do things that feed your body and soul.

If, however, you are in early labor at night, it is a different story. If it's time to be in bed, *do not pass go, do not collect $200*. Go to bed. We know it's hard to sleep when you feel that excited. You'll want to call your mother and your girlfriends. You'll get a second wind and the sudden urge to clear out the lint from the dryer, refold all of your linens, and paint the living room wall a fabulous color of red.

Don't do it. None of it. Zip. Zilch. Nada. As you will read later in this chapter, exhaustion is a major cause for moving from a homebirth to a hospital birth. To avoid that, do the best you can to stick to your normal sleep cycle. Even if you are sleeping for ten or fifteen minutes between contractions, waking up with them, and then resting or drifting off again, you will be in far better shape than trying to pull an all-nighter and chasing that with twenty-four hours of demanding labor.

When should I call my mother, my doula, and the dog-sitter?

EARLY LABOR IS NOT the time to rally your troops. Certainly let any professionals know that things are warming up and you expect to need them in a few hours. However, even though early labor is fun, it's not the time to put on your hostess apron and throw a party. Early contractions can be shy, and tend to vanish when confronted with a lot of people. Wait until your labor is well established before bringing in your support.

We had a lot of people that wanted to be at our birth. We happily invited them all, as we love them and thought it would be great to welcome this baby into our big family. When labor started, I called them and they came. They were their usual selves—and what I normally love about our families. There was a lot of laughter and a lot of food. After several hours I had this strong feeling that I would never have this baby with so much going on around me. I had a talk with my husband, mother, and midwife about my feelings. The midwife shared her experience that babies do come with lots of people around, it can just take longer as it is harder for the mom to go inside of herself and let everything go. My mother was great—she offered to corral the troops and take them to her house, which was about ten minutes away. I remember shaking my head yes and her telling me that she would be back whenever I wanted her—even if it was to meet the baby.

About an hour after they left, I felt everything move to another level. The contractions got really strong and lasted a long time. I birthed our daughter four hours after the house was cleared, supported by my husband, my midwife, and her student (who I really loved!). My family all came back after we were tucked into bed and had enjoyed each other for a while. It was such a happy time, and I am so grateful that I did not let my birth drag out with everyone there because of guilt or fear of asking for what I needed. I credit my midwife with a lot, but her guidance in helping me find my voice in that moment was her greatest gift to us.

—Mari

I'm in labor and it hurts! What can I do?

YOU MAY FEEL PAIN in your lower abdomen, your back, your hips, or a combination of all three. We've heard mothers say that their hair and fingernails hurt! But we have never met a woman who can actually explain the intensity and pain as they really were. We are designed to develop amnesia around the hardest parts. This is why so many doulas and midwives will tell you to "let it go all the way away" at the end of your strongest contractions. Because once they are gone, they are done, and you don't ever have to do them again.

The best part of labor is that half of it is entirely pain-free. Be-

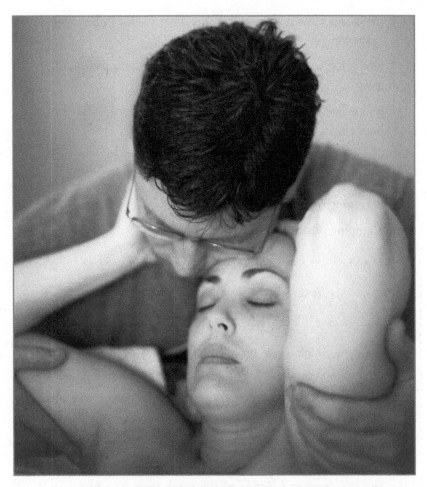

Working hard through active labor.

tween contractions, the goal is to relax completely, quieting your mind and your body. Deep belly-breathing pushes oxygen into your bloodstream, helping to calm the body. Stress and fear make everything worse. If your body is releasing stress hormones like adrenaline, and you do not feel comfortable in your environment, your brain will perceive the pain as being more intense. Homebirthers have an advantage here! People tend to feel the most comfortable in their own homes, surrounded by their people, their pheromones, and their chosen birth team. Here are a few other comfort measures. Most are very simple, but a few require some advance preparation:

- massage: most mothers find this most useful in between contractions
- heat: rice socks, heating pads, and handwarmers are all great
- ice packs: wrap them in a towel first, as they can freeze bare skin
- meditation
- guided imagery
- bouncing on a birth ball
- changing position frequently

Your Autonomic Nervous System: At Work *or* at Play

Can you think of a time when you were panicked? A time when you were fully relaxed? A time when you were working hard but felt calm nonetheless? These states are controlled by your autonomic nervous system, and are important for your birthing experience.

Your autonomic nervous system has two components, and they cannot function at the same time. The first is responsible for your "fight-or-flight" capability and is called your sympathetic nervous system. In the event of danger (perceived or real), your body creates a physical reaction that helps support your emotional one. Your blood is diverted to your muscles and lungs, your heart rate is increased, your pupils will dilate, and your digestive system shuts down. You are primed to survive!

The second is responsible for your "feed-and-breed" or "rest-and-digest" capacity. It is called your parasympathetic nervous system. It opens up the blood flow to your gut, calms your heart, allows you to cry, constricts your pupils for better close-up vision, and stimulates sexual arousal. You are primed to relax and learn, release tension, have awareness of your breath, engage your body, or just enjoy a really good meal with friends.

You cannot be in both states at one time—you have to pick one, and be that. It can change back and forth but it is physiologically impossible to do them both in the same moment. This matters for birthing. You want to keep yourself in the feed-and-breed state and out of the fight-or-flight state for most of labor. If you work with your breath, trusting your body and your baby and all of the sensations they bring to you, you can work really hard *and* stay in your feed-and-breed state. If your body and mind know that your survival isn't threatened, that you are safe and healthy, your labor will proceed smoothly and consistently.

Your well-being should not feel endangered during labor, until you reach what textbooks refer to as transition. Transition occurs as the final 2 centimeters of your cervix are opening up. You receive an internal message to finish up birthing and to do it well. This is when women say the kinds of things that make it into movie scripts: "Why did you do this to me?" "Just cut me open and take it out already!" "I changed my mind!" "You'll never touch me again as long as I live!" And our favorite: "I can't do it anymore!" Why is that our favorite? Because we know that when a woman screams this, "I can't do it anymore," it's because she can't. She is almost done. Her sympathetic nervous system kicks into high gear, and her senses come alive in new ways as everything about her prepares to birth her baby in the very near future.

Knowing how your autonomic nervous system works provides a valuable tool for responding to your labor. Use this knowledge to maintain awareness of what state you are in, especially during early and middle labor. If you are the kind of person who tends toward panic, use your pregnancy to practice calming techniques with your partner. You can then use these together if you start to feel anxiety creeping up during labor.

I've heard position changes can be really helpful for comfort during labor. Can you give me some examples?

IF WE HAD TO choose the most important factor in a woman's labor, it would be the ability to move freely. Think of your labor as a dance between you and your baby. A good dance partner telegraphs how you should move. Imagine those elderly couples you see dancing at weddings, the ones who get back on the floor after the Funky Chicken. They seem ethereal in the way their bodies communicate. This is precisely what happens between you and your baby. Your baby moves one way, and you will instinctively move in a complementary manner. It can be hard to remember that your baby is an active participant in your labor, but she most certainly is. She is doing her best, just as you are! The best position is the one that feels right to you in the moment. When it doesn't feel right anymore, move.

Positional changes can turn a baby, straighten out her head, or fix an abnormal heart rate. They can open your pelvis and make the pain more bearable. They are every woman's friend, and every midwife's secret weapon. Many, many women have said that they cannot imagine having their movements restricted during labor.

I think my labor would have hurt more in the hospital. I spent such a huge chunk of labor crawling around on my carpet on my hands and knees. It was the only way I could stand it, as I had massive back labor. I was also sleeping in between contractions and that would have been much less comfortable and very unsanitary on the hospital floor (if they would have even allowed it)!

—Zoe

Can you tell me about waterbirth?

WATERBIRTH IS A VERY popular option for homebirthers. A large tub full of warm water has been called the midwife's epidural. It provides significant pain relief, as the warm water soothes and relaxes tired muscles. Many women use the tub intermittently throughout labor, while others stay in straight through.

It is easy to change positions using the water to move in. Kneeling, hands and knees, semi-reclining, and a variety of yoga positions are all popular in the water. If your tub is big enough for two, many partners love to join the mother in the water. It can be extremely relaxing, resting comfortably in your partner's arms.

Sometimes a regular bath tub is large enough, but often a woman enjoys the freedom of movement afforded by a larger pool. There are several types available for purchase or for rent. We have found the large inflatable pools to be quite comfortable. They are inflated on the bottom as well as the sides, so they are cushy on the knees. They also often have an inflatable "step" on the inside that mothers like to sit on, and come with convenient disposable liners. All tubs are filled initially using a hose and all of the hot water your tank will provide. We then add cold water to get to the right temperature. They have no heaters, but we've never had a problem getting a dad to boil a pot of water to add in to keep the temperature up where it needs to be.

I love hot baths. How hot can the birth tub be?

WE'VE FOUND OVER THE years that the best temperature for birthing is between 96 and 98 degrees. You are working hard, so any hotter than that, and you can easily become dehydrated, lethargic, and exhausted. If you get overheated, your baby's heart rate increases to higher-than-normal rates and your midwife will get you out of the tub to cool you both down. Our rules for waterbirth success are these:

- Keep the temperature between 96 and 98 degrees Fahrenheit.

- Drink between 1 and 2 quarts of fluids for every hour you are in the water. We prefer fluid with a kick to it—so add something like grape juice, apple juice, or electrolytes to your water. A sports drink or coconut water are also great options.

- Stay in the water for one hour, get out for thirty minutes. This keeps your temperature even and allows you time to move in different ways. The big bonus is that after staying out of the water for a half hour, every time you get back in, you will feel the relief of escaping gravity all over again!

My mother wants to know why the baby doesn't try to breathe underwater.

THIS IS A VERY common question. It does seem a little counterintuitive. However, once people remember that babies are actually living in water the whole time they are inside of their moms, it makes more sense. Additionally, babies who are born underwater are not left there—they are brought up to the surface and to their mother's chest right away.

Your baby continues to get her oxygen needs met through her umbilical cord even after she is born. It takes time for babies to transition from water-breathing (as in the womb) to air-breathing (as in your

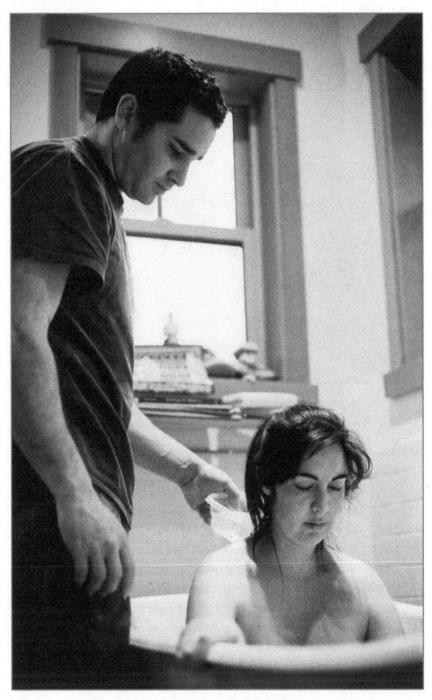

Water helps soothe intense labor contractions.

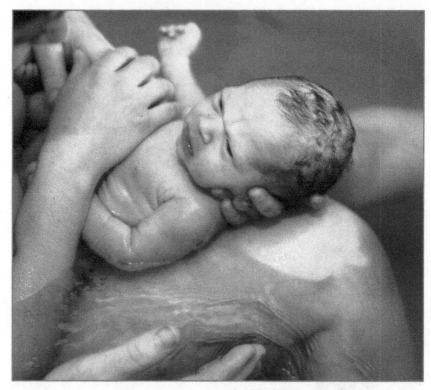

Welcoming baby after a warm and gentle waterbirth.

living room). There is usually more than enough time to take the baby out of the water before it takes its first breath.

> I absolutely cannot imagine having a baby on land. My first son's birth was one of the highlights of my entire life. I had labored hard, for about fourteen hours, and had actually forgotten that I even had the tub! When my midwife reminded me about it, I didn't even want to get in. It just seemed like too much trouble. But when I got in . . . AHHHHHHHH. Sweet relief. It didn't take all the pain away, far from it, but it let me relax completely in between contractions, so I could float and rest. It was amazing. I felt like I could finally concentrate on actually having a baby. And a couple of hours later, I did!
>
> —Laurel

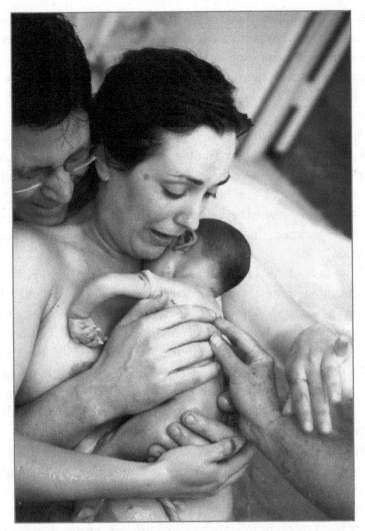

The first joyous seconds shared with mom, dad, and baby.

Do you have any other ideas to make my labor as effective as it can be?

RELEASE IS THE NAME of the game. When you kick into active labor, let the rest fall away. Let go of everything: worry over your partner's experience, to-do lists, whether or not you *look* like a laboring mother. We've seen moms stop their labor because they could not let go of their upper, thinking mind. This is the result of hormones that are designed to protect our species, going way back to when our foremothers were birthing in the wild. If a laboring mom sensed or recognized a threat, her body would flood with chemicals that would stop the labor. This allowed her to hightail it to a safer place to continue her birth.

Today if you sense trouble, it will probably not be a bear or a war party causing you difficulty. Trouble for homebirth moms now usually comes in the form of a toddler. Moms will be puttering through labor all day and then kick into high gear as soon as the siblings are put to bed. When they know they're safe from having to meet the needs of their older children, they are able to let themselves get into strong active labor.

Trouble for homebirth moms also comes in the form of *control*. Homebirthing women today are usually educated, and may have worked in a setting where they manage people, divisions, or whole corporations. They rely on timecards, hard data, and collaboration with others as tools to get through their day successfully. Even mothers who don't work outside the home tend to have highly scheduled lives, particularly when other children are involved. When it comes to birth and parenting, that all goes out the window. When we birth and mother, we are returning to our primitive selves.

We are down to the biology of what makes us who we are. You will be surrounded by those who love you and those you have invited to attend you, but you will be isolated within your experience. You are the only one who can birth this baby. Embrace this moment for what it is—a moment to surrender to a process greater than yourself, a moment to listen to your body, a moment to release all of the outside voices and follow your own inner guidance system.

How will I know when it is time to push?

EVEN IF YOU WERE birthing alone in a cave, eventually you would feel the overwhelming urge to push. It is unmistakable. Even your hair and toenails want to push.

Some mothers enter the pushing stage gradually. They feel a lot of rectal pressure at the peak of each contraction. As their bodies dilate the last 2 centimeters or so, this pressure builds until the feelings associated with dilating are taken over by the sensation of pressure and fullness, and you can do nothing else except push.

Other times there will be a break in the contractions for a few minutes, when the body has finished dilating and is gearing up to push. This allows for restoration of strength and focus. Many mothers fall asleep during this time. And not just any little cat nap, but a nectar-of-the-gods kind of sleep as your body gathers energy for the coming effort. There is often snoring involved. Other mothers get ravenously hungry and pause in their labor for some serious chow time. Again, this is the body's way of building up that reserve of strength needed for birth.

Will my midwife check me to be sure it's okay to push?

WE FEEL THAT A vaginal exam is one of many tools a midwife can use when it comes to gathering information about a mother's labor. Each midwife practices differently, and every mother has a different comfort level when it comes to vaginal exams, so it's a good idea to chat about the frequency of exams prenatally to avoid surprises. Vaginal exams give you a snapshot of how dilated you are at that particular moment, but they aren't predictive of how your labor will unfold. If you are 7 centimeters dilated, you may stay that way for another five hours or you may be pushing out your baby in fifteen minutes. There is no way to tell.

Each exam includes increased risk of infection, particularly if your water has broken. And there is always the danger that your team could superimpose onto your birth their ideas about how fast or slow you are moving along. Additionally, there is usually some discomfort with these exams.

There are many signs that a woman is moving forward in her labor and birthing. The sounds, smells, and a variety of sights are familiar markers along the path for an experienced birthing professional. Your intuitive sense of the changes in your body should provide the most important information for you and for your midwife. You will eventually experience that absolutely overwhelming need to bear down along with your contractions. Everyone around you will hear and feel the difference as you move into this phase of labor.

What will pushing feel like?

MOST PEOPLE CALL IT the most surreal experience of their lives. Many women report that pushing feels good, or at least better than dilating. This is likely because, after hours of working to release your tension and allow the baby to move down, you finally get to participate in an active way.

Is there a special way to breathe when I am pushing?

NO. YOU HAVE BEEN breathing effectively since the moment you came into this world. When you run, you breathe faster or deeper, and when you are standing in line at the grocery store, you chest or belly breathe. During labor, there are often long, deep breaths between pushes. This occurs quite naturally; it's your body's way of pulling in oxygen, so the red blood cells can distribute it to all of the parts of your and your baby's bodies. There is no right or wrong way to breath. Your midwife or doula will cue you if it looks like you are holding your breath or breathing too quickly. Other than that, follow your body and fill your lungs in whatever way feels good.

Can my body actually birth without splitting in two?

YES. WE PROMISE. AS your baby moves down the birth canal, you will feel intense pressure. Your tissues and the ligaments joining your bones are made to stretch and give. They are extra loose during pregnancy and labor from an increase in the hormone called relaxin. This is the hormone that makes you clutzy, waddle when you walk, and drop things all of the time. It also allows your pelvis to get some 30 percent bigger than it is normally. Some women like a warm wet compress applied to their perineum during this time to soothe that skin as it stretches. As your baby's head starts to crown (when the widest part of your baby's head is born), you will feel the "ring of fire." This burning/stretching sensation only lasts through the next contraction, when the head is fully out, and many women look forward to this as a signal that they're almost finished.

Who will catch my baby?

THIS IS ONE OF the delights of midwifery care for many families. You are welcome to catch your baby into your own hands, or Dad, Grandma, or an older sibling can! Your midwife will likely put her hands under whoever's hands are there, as babies are a bit slippery when they are so freshly arrived.

Is there anything I can do to prevent having to transfer to the hospital?

IT'S IMPORTANT TO KNOW that most women do not transfer their care from home to hospital in an ambulance with sirens wailing. But if they do change locations, it is usually because of the length of the labor and subsequent exhaustion. Midwives all over the world are familiar with the woman who goes into labor around 11:00 p.m., does not sleep through the early contractions, and then labors through the following day. By the next night, her body is just too tired to birth safely at home. Take the steps to avoid exhaustion. And it is worth saying again, in case you are lying in bed with infrequent yet regular contractions right now . . . your body will wake you up when it really needs you to participate in this labor. So, lights out and sweet dreams!

What are some situations in which I might have to transfer?

- fatigue
- pain management
- maternal fever or high blood pressure
- significant blood loss prior to the birth
- baby's heart rate too low or too high (and not resolved using the many techniques your midwife will try)
- meconium in the amniotic fluid
- uncontrolled postpartum hemorrhage
- retained placentas (a placenta that does not separate from the uterine wall)
- newborns who cannot maintain their temperature
- newborn anomalies that require pediatric care

The Midwife Says: Meconium is baby's first poop. It's black and sticky and you can probably tar roofs with it. Meconium can be of concern if the baby poops before she is born. When inhaled, it can cause a rare respiratory syndrome requiring medical treatment. A study of almost 3,500 newborns showed that the presence of meconium in the amniotic fluid does not change outcomes for babies.[6] It has to occur with other factors (such as a compromised heart rate) to be a warning sign that a baby may need extra support. If your baby decides to poop en utero, your midwife will talk with you about your options.

I think I need to transfer to the hospital. How can I talk about this and how do women feel who do it?

IF YOU FEEL SOMETHING is not right during your labor or the post-partum time, tell your midwife. Talk about what you feel needs attention. We value intuition in a very big way and can help put together the pieces of your puzzle by asking questions, eliminating certain conditions, and gathering more information. If, for any reason, you feel you and/or your baby might benefit from a hospital visit, please share this information with your midwife. We know mothers who transferred for something they couldn't quite quantify, who did indeed wind up needing specialized care. Trust your feelings. We do.

If you are transferred to the hospital, it is because you need something you didn't have access to at home. If this is the case, you have already done all you could do to have your homebirth. Your team believes there are good reasons to seek specialized care. The midwifery model of care is not about preventing the need for a hospital birth. It is about using appropriate resources to keep you and your baby healthy.

Homebirth transfers are not "failed homebirths." The use of hospital care does not invalidate the investment you made in yourself, your family, and your baby throughout pregnancy and labor.

> When I look back on my birth, I have so many conflicting feelings. I felt hurt and sad when my homebirth did not turn out as I had planned. But I also see how very hard I tried and I cannot think of a thing I could or should have done differently. My midwife patiently helped me come to this realization. Her postpartum support was wonderful. Even though Matthew was born at the hospital, she came to the house for all of my postpartum checks, and I went to her for my 8-week appointment.
>
> —Carla

The Midwife Says: After a transfer to the hospital, regardless of the reason, we have found two things really help a mother process and understand her experience. The first is to have someone from our team go with the mother and stay in the hospital with her through delivery. The second is to pick up with postpartum care at home when she returns. We keep the same schedule and use the time to listen to her birth story as well as provide information she wants. If she has a copy of her chart from the hospital, we read it together.

We love on her and the baby exactly the way we would have had she birthed at home. We teach self-attachment for breastfeeding if Mom and Baby didn't try it in the hospital. (Babies are always ready and willing to show off their amazing skills!) If she needs extra support, we give it without question. It is important to celebrate and honor the full and actual experiences mothers have, and this applies to our planned-homebirth, delivered-in-the-hospital mamas too!

I did it! I had a homebirth!

IN THE MOMENTS AND days just after birth, it is our wish that mothers coo and admire not just their babies but their own prowess and powers that brought them through their pregnancy, labor, and birthing. Midwives never want to be the heroines of your story; we thrive when mothers thrive in their own abilities and recognize the resilience and strength that exist deep inside of them. Look to yourself for your knowledge and courage; they are there, always a part of you. Birth will showcase this truth in ways that will profoundly affect the rest of your life as a mother and woman.

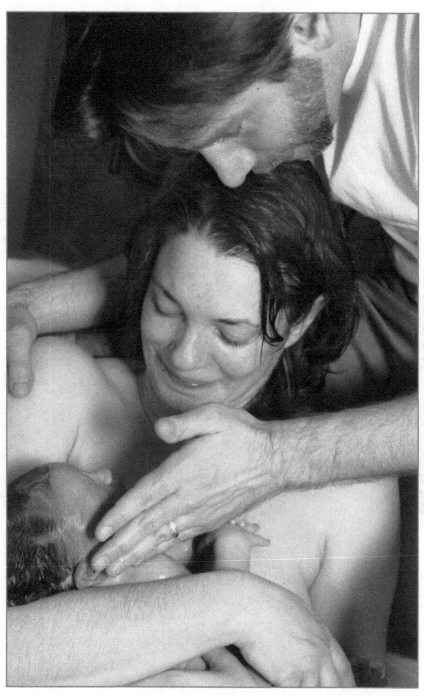

These parents greet their new baby for the first time.

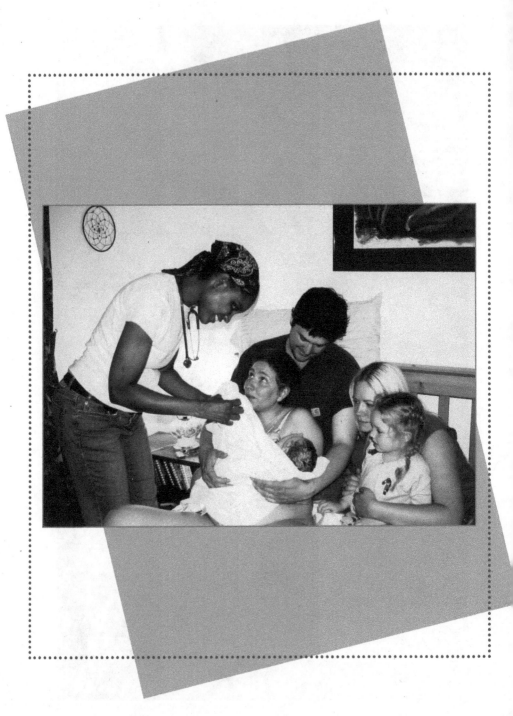

CHAPTER ELEVEN

The Postpartum Period

- Immediate postpartum care
- Skin-to-skin
- Breastfeeding your baby
- What's next?
- Newborn medications and screening
- Postpartum depression

MAMA SAYS

Near the end of my third pregnancy, one of my requests to my midwife was to remind me to spend some time with the baby, to just be wet and warm, connected, and free to just be with each other. And that's what I remember. I remember holding a baby girl, which was a surprise. I remember spending time looking at her and wondering how she could look so much like our first son. I remember the placenta being delivered and my middle son cutting the cord. While I don't remember many more particular moments, I remember feeling good. Relieved. I loved that it was just my little family around me and there was nowhere we needed to go.

—Courtney

Immediate Postpartum Care

YOU'VE DELIVERED, AND ALL is well. Now what happens? Your midwife has work to do during this time to ensure Mom and Baby are healthy and doing well. In the first four hours, there is a lot of loving and bonding and many care-plan decisions to make. Just like during pregnancy, there is no "right" way to act or feel directly after the birth of a child. The options available for care vary depending on you, your baby, and the choices you make.

How is my baby cared for just after birth?

WHILE YOU MAY HAVE plenty of images in your head from movies and TV of babies being whisked off to incubators, midwives know that

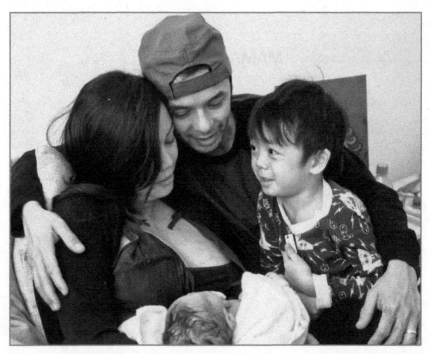

An entire family together, meeting its newest member.

mothers, not plastic boxes, are their baby's natural habitat. Babies will do their best in your arms and when their umbilical cords are kept intact. You can expect that your baby will be placed on your chest and that we will observe her in a variety of ways to ensure her well-being. We watch for signs that she is breathing well and that she has a good heart rate. When those two systems are working well, it usually indicates that the baby is healthy.

Can you tell me more about keeping the umbilical cord intact? I thought it had to be cut right away.

THE UMBILICAL CORD IS the conduit for nutrient- and oxygen-rich blood to go to the baby and for waste products to be eliminated from the baby's bloodstream. During pregnancy you can imagine a figure eight system, cycling in the good and taking away the bad. At any given time, about one-third of the baby's blood supply is in the placenta, on the other end of the figure eight. When one feels the cord after birth, it has a pulse to it. This pulse is the signal that the body is still running blood through that figure eight. At the time of birth, the amount of blood in the baby is decided upon by a power far beyond our control. A natural homeostasis is reached in which your baby will have just the right amount of blood that he needs. At that time, which can range from a few minutes to more than twenty minutes, you will be able to feel the cord "stop pulsing." Most homebirth midwives have been doing this for years, and it is becoming more and more popular in the hospital as well. Keeping the cord intact is also known as delayed cord clamping. This term can refer either to waiting for the cord to stop pulsing or simply waiting thirty seconds to three minutes after birth before cutting the cord. Be sure to talk with your midwife about her practice and what your wishes are.

There is some very good science around delayed cord clamping in regards to anemia in babies. These include

- HIGHER INFANT HEMOGLOBIN LEVELS (Hemoglo-
  bin is a protein molecule in red blood cells that transports

oxygen from the lungs to body tissues. Higher hemoglobin levels=higher oxygenation.) [1]

- HIGHER INFANT FERRITIN LEVELS (Ferritin is another protein. This one stores iron, and releases it in a controlled fashion. One Mexican study showed an increase of total iron stores of up to 47 milligrams!) [2]

- HIGHER INFANT HEMATOCRITS AND BLOOD PRESSURES [3] (The hematocrit levels reflect the percentage of the baby's blood that is occupied by red blood cells, while the blood pressure measurement is a good indicator of how efficiently the heart is pumping.)

What happens to my placenta?

FIRST YOU GET TO meet it! The placenta is often the unsung hero of the birthing process. Just imagine, you've grown an entire organ over the course of your pregnancy. It supplies your baby with oxygen and nourishment, allowing her to grow to her fullest potential. And then, when you don't need it anymore, it slides out. It's the body's only completely disposable organ. We are true placenta fans.

We encourage you to examine your placenta. Have your midwife point out which side was attached to your uterine wall and where the umbilical cord was implanted. Check out the two arteries and one vein inside the cord. You can see them clearly. Have her hold up the broken amniotic sac, so you can see the little apartment your baby lived in for nine months. Examine the intricate array of blood vessels on the fetal side, called the Tree of Life. Some women take a moment to thank the placenta for its work.

Some homebirth families have developed meaningful rituals around their placentas. Many bury them under a special tree. (Dig a deep hole. Animals also love placentas!) Others choose to encapsulate it. This process involves drying the placenta, crushing it, and then putting it into capsules. Proponents of this claim that the pills are good for postpartum depression, or, later on, for managing the effects

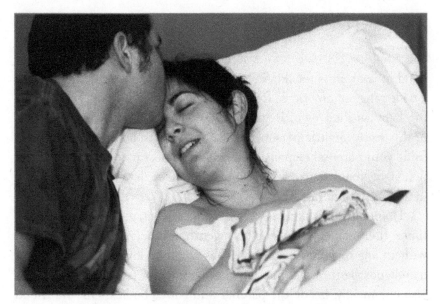

The first moments postpartum are the sweetest.

of menopause. We haven't seen any good research on this, but we encourage everyone to follow their hearts. If you do not wish to hold on to your placenta, your midwife will take it with her and dispose of it.

My baby is the most beautiful baby in the world! Have you ever seen a baby so cute?

IT'S FASCINATING TO WATCH a mother discover her baby for the first time. Left completely undisturbed, most mammals follow a distinct pattern, and humans are no exception. They won't pick up the baby right away. Instead, they slowly touch the baby, starting with the extremities, and then work their way in toward the heart. Then the mother will swoop the baby into her arms. She will slowly smell the baby's head, nuzzle, and hold the baby at breast height.

How can I encourage bonding?

THERE IS NOTHING MORE intense and profound than holding your child in your arms for the first time. Both mothers and fathers report a wide range of emotions, from euphoric bliss to not even recognizing the baby as their own. Regardless of what your initial impression is of this squiggly little person, you will be able to bond with them and fulfill your parental responsibilities. While most parents report love at first sight, many take a few minutes, hours, or days to completely fall in love with their new baby.

Homebirthing families do have an advantage. The majority of times, their babies have been born gently, on their own timetable, and without any major interventions. This creates a lovely scenario immediately postpartum, not just environmentally for postbirth photos but also chemically, inside the parents' and baby's bodies. Our old friend oxytocin is at work again.

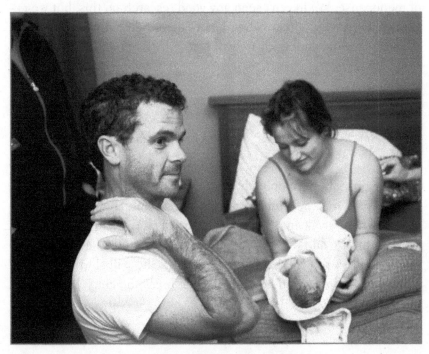

This mama counts fingers and toes.

How does oxytocin help immediately postpartum?

OXYTOCIN, YOU MAY REMEMBER, is known as the love hormone, as it is responsible for all those lovey-dovey feelings new parents specialize in. During an ideal birth, this hormone ebbs and flows as needed, in exactly the right amounts. This not only results in excellent contractions but allows the birthing mother to feel deeply connected to everyone around her. Most mothers remember everyone in the room with love and a dreamy fondness. Women in this state are also highly suggestible. Their hearts are wide open, and so should be treated with the utmost gentleness and respect.

In fact, by the time the baby joins us, everyone in the room is usually bathing in oxytocin! We all have it. Watching a mother birth can be profound; most people experience it only a few times. Birth professionals often speak of a "birth high," an altered euphoric state we tend to experience after a particularly rewarding night. In fact, it could be one of the reasons we love our jobs so much! And of course, it is a special joy to watch a man become a father, whether it is for the first time or the fourteenth. The combination of tenderness, awe, and protectiveness is magical and sacred. His oxytocin receptors are working in high gear, setting him up for a lifetime of loving his family.

Skin-to-Skin

I keep hearing about something called skin-to-skin. What is it?

IF WE LEFT YOU alone to birth, you would naturally bring your baby up to your chest in the first minutes after birth. This connecting of the new baby to the mother is as old as time. As technology grew, we became separated from skin-to-skin contact. The warm body and loving arms of a mother were replaced with warming lights in nurseries for healthy babies and incubators for babies born too early or ill.

However, when two doctors tried to solve an incubator-shortage in Bogota, Columbia, in 1979 using skin-to-skin care, their results were very positive.[4]

In the mid-1980s, research started to pour in, showing skin-to-skin care led to better outcomes than the use of incubators. Dr. Nils Bergman introduced this care for use in the NICU with premature babies in South Africa. Known in the NICU as "Kangaroo Mother Care," it includes skin-to-skin contact, breastfeeding, and adding technology to this physical arrangement *when necessary*. This was a very different care plan than the standard one, which relied primarily on technological caregiving and allowed only infrequent physical connection between the mother and baby. The research showed that Kangaroo Mother Care babies were warmer and calmer, breathed better, and had a more stable heart rate due to skin-to-skin care.[5] Healthy babies enjoy all of the same benefits. Additionally, because they are stable physically, they are able to engage emotionally and intellectually with their mothers and the world around them.

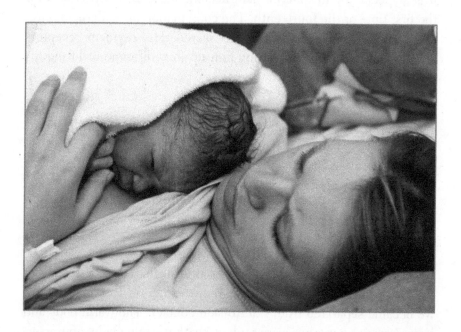

What are the benefits for the baby of skin-to-skin positioning after birth?

WHILE BABIES ARE BORN with skills to help ensure their survival, such as state regulation (the ability to protect their sleep and move from sleep to wake to fussy and back again smoothly) and self-attachment (the ability to self-latch onto the breast), they are also extremely dependent upon their mothers to provide the support and environment where these skills can be put to use. For example, babies will naturally root, opening their mouths and turning their heads so that they can feed. A baby does this when she is hungry but it is the mother who, present and holding her baby, will feel these movements and naturally make the breast available for her child. A baby who is fed on demand has an easy connection between its behavior and the response it receives.

This idea of the mother and baby as deeply interconnected beings is the reason they are often referred to as the mother/baby dyad.

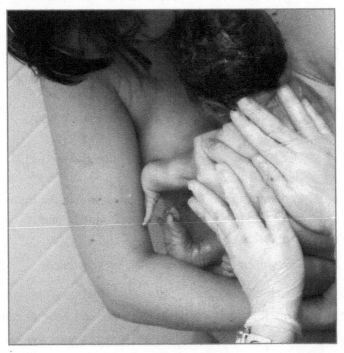

Skin-to-skin contact has many positive effects for both mom and baby.

What is done to or for one will always affect the other. Your baby's temperature, heart rate, and breathing rate will all regulate faster and smoother if your baby is placed skin-to-skin with you immediately after birth. Research has shown that no less than one hour of this contact is necessary, but ongoing skin-to-skin contact is extremely beneficial through the first day and into the early weeks of life.[6]

Help Wanted

If we could write a job description for your baby from birth through the first few weeks of life, it would read:

Position Available: *Super Adorable Newborn Baby*

Requirements:

- ★ Stay warm.
- ★ Ingest calories with proper mix of nutrients for developing gut.
- ★ Maintain regulation of heart rate, respiratory rate, and brain development.
- ★ Grow much faster than you ever will in your entire life again.
- ★ Digestive capabilities a must: urinate and poop many times per day.
- ★ Use behavior to communicate needs, likes, and dislikes.
- ★ Look mother and father in the eye and make them smile and laugh through use of imitation and expressions of curiosity.

Salary: Room, board, and eventually an allowance

That is a big job for such a little baby! The benefit of skin-to-skin contact is that it reduces this workload. Mother can take a lot off of the baby's plate and make the rest a whole

---

lot easier just by holding her baby next to her. A mother's chest adjusts and will warm if a baby is too cold or cool if a baby is too warm. Breast milk production is helped by the closeness of Baby, producing the nourishment he needs for a great start in life. Baby gains exposure to the multitude of germs on Mom's body, which helps develop his immune system. Skin-to-skin frees a healthy baby from a multitude of tasks and allows her to use her energy for higher growth.

Doesn't so much holding spoil the baby right from the start?

NO. BUT ANY DISCONNECT between the baby's behavior and the response he gets from you can create challenges for him as he grows. A child who trusts himself starts as a baby who is felt and heard and responded to by his parents. Spoiling implies a rotting from within. Responding to Baby's cues and fulfilling that role of environmental support builds strength, trust, and confidence at the core of a child. Baby's very substance is the opposite of rot, which occurs with neglect, not with care. Research has shown that babies who are neglected stop trying to engage. They stop their inborn behaviors, which demonstrate need, and the core of what makes us human—seeking relationships with others—evaporates.[7]

Holding your baby close to you, so that her ear is on your heart, helps regulate her most basic needs: an even heart rate, smooth breath, and a temperature that allows for optimal health. It also frames her world in the love and understanding you have for who she is and what her needs will be.

Are there benefits of skin-to-skin care for me?

YES, THERE ARE! SKIN-TO-SKIN care releases oxytocin, which calms and soothes you and helps with the production of breast milk. Your baby has easy access to the breast and may start sucking soon after birth or within the first hour or two. As your baby nurses, hormones are released, helping the uterus to contract, which limits blood loss. Your baby will regulate himself to your rhythms—and will often even sleep when you sleep. This synchronicity that exists between Mother and Baby stays finely tuned as long as you commit to being still with him.

We like our mothers to commit to a full week in bed after birth. This allows for optimal physical healing and for the important resetting of a mother's rhythms so that she syncs with her baby. Babies move slowly. A mother's work in the first moments and days of life is to become attuned to this pace. After years of schooling and employment, management responsibilities, deadlines, and early-morning rush-hour races to work, life comes to a sluggish, slow-moving pace.

This can be quite shocking for many mothers, but we have found that once this adjustment is made, they find great joy and liberation in

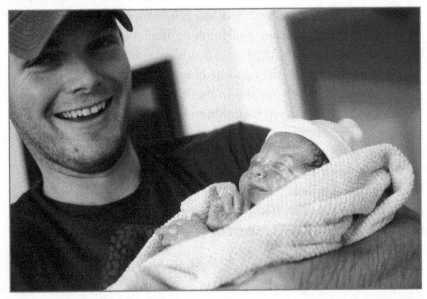

Big smiles from Dad.

The Postpartum Period   283

just being with the baby. This time isn't called a babymoon for nothing! It can be hard to prepare for, but keep in mind that your best health will come with lying low and keeping your baby close.

If there is some kind of emergency and I am separated from my baby, have I ruined our chances of proper bonding?

ABSOLUTELY NOT. THAT BEARS saying again: absolutely not. Babies and mothers are much more resilient than that. If you are separated from your baby, he will benefit from skin-to-skin care during the moments you can provide it, from whenever you start it. Babies are programmed not only to survive but to thrive, and this is the perfect showcase for them. If there is a physical emergency with you, such as postpartum hemorrhage, then your body is not in a normal postpartum state anyway. It needs some help before it can respond hormonally and chemically in an optimum way. Babies need their autonomic system—the breathing and heart function—to be fully functioning before they become available for the emotional work of bonding and relationship. So if your baby needs extra care right after birth, do not worry about missed moments, or even days. Once everyone is stable, the bonding will begin and you will flourish as a team from that point forward.

Breastfeeding Your Baby

What should I know about breastfeeding?

THERE ARE WONDERFUL BOOKS that cover breastfeeding in detail, and we highly recommend reading one or two as you prepare to nurse your baby. Additionally, attending a prenatal breastfeeding class can give you access to the basic tools, language, and resources unique to breastfeeding.

It takes time for a mom and baby to find the position that works for them, and there is no one right way to breastfeed your baby. Be patient with yourself and with your baby, and don't be discouraged if you don't master this process right away—it is normal and fine to have to work on it. The early postpartum time is wonderful for exploring each other and helping the baby fall in love with the breast as he finds comfort just being close to you.

If you have questions or want guidance or help with breastfeeding, contact your local La Leche League chapter or search for an IBCLC (discussed at length in chapter six).

Is there a position that generally works well for first-time nursing moms?

FINDING THE RIGHT POSITION might take several tries or you may get it on the first go. Start by getting comfortable: use lots of pillows under your arms, behind you, and underneath the baby to provide good support. Here are some basic position ideas:

- Position your knees higher than your hips
- Place your baby at the level of your nipples
- Baby's chest, belly, and knees should all touch your abdomen
- Baby should be faced so that he is looking at your nipple, and does not have to turn his head toward it while feeding
- Baby's ear, shoulder, and hip should be in one straight line
- When you sit slightly reclined by leaning back on some pillows, the baby stays in a great nursing position with very little effort

How will I know when it is time to nurse my baby?

BABIES WHO ARE READY to eat use their behavior to communicate this need. These behaviors can cue Mom to offer the breast:

- Baby puts his hand in his mouth and turns his head toward the side

- Baby turns his head to one side and opens his mouth (this is called "rooting")

- Baby will suck on anything he can

- Babies may be awake or asleep when they exhibit these behaviors. All are normal and healthy and indicate hunger.

How will I know when my baby has had enough breast milk?

BABIES NATURALLY PULL AWAY from the breast when they are finished. If you support the head and neck without applying pressure, you will feel the baby pull back. A baby who is full does not exhibit any of the behaviors listed here that demonstrate hunger.

Molly Pessl, BN, IBCLC, offers these tips for breastfeeding:

- Feed early, feed often.

- Keep your baby next to your skin for the first hours.

- Early postpartum is a learning time for you and your baby. Stay patient with yourself and your baby; it will work but sometimes it takes a bit of time!

- Limit visitors (especially in the first few hours after birth) to protect the unique postpartum environment.

- Don't count the number of feedings or overanalyze your baby's nursing schedule. Just feed him whenever he seems interested. He knows what to do!

- Your baby does not know how to read a clock, so nursing (like so much of newborn life) is not time-bound. Allow him to nurse as long as he wants to.

- The more your baby nurses in the first few days, the better. Not only does he master his technique, but he is helping to establish a good supply for the coming days and months.

- Even one bottle of formula alters the entire Ph balance of the baby's stomach and gut.

- If you are having problems, keep working on the breastfeeding and ask for support.

What's Next?

How do I know my baby is healthy?

YOUR MIDWIFE WILL DO a thorough exam of your baby, after you have had time to bond and nurse. She will check for any abnormalities in his physical structure, be sure that he is neurologically intact, and do the all-important measuring and weighing. All of this should be performed on the bed next to you, and everything should be explained to you as it is done.

If I need stitches, how does that work?

YOUR MIDWIFE WILL CHECK to see if your perineum has torn during the birth. If so, she will assess the laceration, and if she feels it needs stitches, will do the repair. Some homebirth midwives are not allowed to suture according to their state's law. It's a good idea to talk

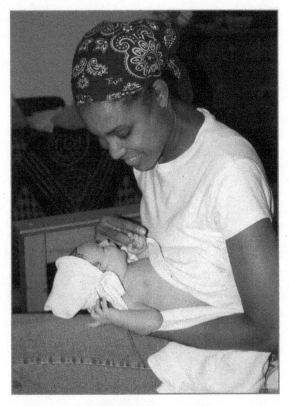

A midwife welcomes Baby.

about this prenatally. If you have torn badly, you may need to transfer to the hospital to get some help. This is unlikely at a homebirth, as you are encouraged to push just as your body tells you, but it does happen.

I really don't want to be alone right away; when does the midwife leave?

WE DON'T WANT YOU to be alone, either! Most midwives routinely stay between three and five hours after a birth. We want to be sure that you and your baby are stable, and that all is well. If there have been any complications, we will stay even longer. Throughout the immediate postpartum period, your midwife will take your vital signs,

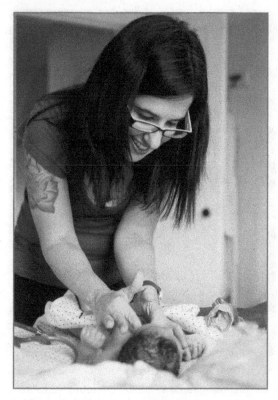

A midwife performing a complete newborn examination.

watch your baby, and make sure you are not bleeding too much. She will massage your uterus to expel any clots, making sure your bleeding is controlled. If you received any medications during the birth, such as Pitocin or misoprostol, she will want to be sure they have completely cleared your body and that your bleeding is well controlled. If you had an IV for any reason, she will remove it before she leaves.

Eventually you will get up to urinate, and if you feel up to it, take a quick shower. While you are attending to these tasks, your midwife will change your sheets, tidy the room, and make you something to eat. Giving birth is hungry work. There's just nothing nicer than coming back to a fresh room, eating a home-cooked meal, and snuggling with your baby. When your midwife is sure that you and your baby are stable, she will gather her things together, offer instructions for the first twenty-four hours of care for you and Baby, and take her leave.

Newborn Medications and Screening

Can you tell me about vitamin K?

ALL BABIES BORN IN the United States are offered an injection of vitamin K at birth. The standard protocols say this is to prevent a disorder called Vitamin K Deficiency Bleeding (VKDB). (It used to be known as hemorrhagic disease of the newborn.) Your baby uses vitamin K to help make clotting factors, substances that prevent excessive bleeding. If he is lacking these factors, and internal or external bleeding occurs, it can be serious.

What exactly is VKDB? Are there situations that predispose my baby to have it?

VKDB IS DEFINED AS internal or external bleeding in newborns, not associated with trauma, accident, or hereditary bleeding disorders.[8] There are three types. The first is early-onset VKDB, where bleeding begins within the first twenty-four hours of birth. It is extremely rare, and usually happens when the mother has taken drugs to control epilepsy during her pregnancy. Classic-onset VKDB occurs within the first week of birth. The bleeding usually shows up in the intestines, the nose, or the umbilical site. Late-onset VKDB happens after the first week, up to four months or so. In this case, the bleeding is usually in the brain.

There is actually a bit of controversy as to whether low levels of vitamin K actually cause VKDB. Certainly vitamin K stops bleeding. However, that does not necessarily mean that a lack of vitamin K is the cause of this condition. Aspirin cures headaches, but a lack of it in our bodies does not cause them. Some studies on VKDB have found babies with this condition who are not vitamin K deficient at all.[9]

There are certain conditions that are risk factors for VKDB. These include cystic fibrosis, chronic diarrhea, bile duct atresia, celiac disease, and hepatitis. All of these conditions make it difficult for your baby to use or absorb vitamin K.[10] A difficult birth, where your baby arrives a bit bruised and battered, can also increase her chance of VKDB.

My baby does not have any of these conditions. Does she need vitamin K?

ONLY YOU CAN DECIDE this. The risk of your baby getting VKDB is low, but it can be serious. All the statistics in the world do not mean anything when it is your baby. Talk with your midwife, do your research, and access your intuition. Use the BRAINS acronym, discussed in chapter six. And in the end, you will have made a fair, informed choice.

I understand that there is eye medication for newborns. What is this and why is it used?

IT IS AN ANTIBIOTIC ointment called either tetracycline or erythromycin and it is used to prevent an infection in your baby's eyes from exposure to gonorrhea.

How can my baby get gonorrhea in its eyes?

A GONORRHEA INFECTION IN the baby's eyes occurs when a mother has this infection on her cervix or in her vaginal area, and the bacteria are transmitted to the baby during or after birth. If the mother does not have gonorrhea, the baby cannot get it.

How do I know if I have gonorrhea?

A MOTHER OR HER partner can contract gonorrhea before, during, or after pregnancy. Either could contract it from a partner who engaged in sexual activity (vaginal, oral, or anal) with someone who has gonorrhea. The symptoms are not always obvious and for some women there are no outward symptoms at all. If a woman's partner is having sexual relationships with other people, she is at high risk for sexually transmitted infections (STIs), including gonorrhea.

Your midwife can run tests to check you for a variety of STIs. Chlamydia can also cause eye infections for babies, but the infection is typically not as serious as one caused by gonorrhea. Of course every STI comes with a host of symptoms and health consequences. Your midwife will have a detailed discussion with you about these, including testing and treatment options.

What are the benefits of antibiotic treatment in the eyes?

- IT PROVIDES COVERAGE FOR HIGH-RISK MOTHERS: Mothers who are unsure of their own or their partner's sexual history (including during the current pregnancy) have an increased risk of carrying and transmitting gonococcal bacteria. This treatment prevents the transmission of gonorrhea to newborn babies.

- IT ADDRESSES UNCERTAINTIES RESULTING FROM LACK OF PRENATAL CARE: Mothers who did not have standard prenatal screening might not know if they carry the bacteria. They can spare their baby from an aggressive eye infection and prevent the permanent blindness that this infection causes by electing to use this treatment option.

- Providers concerned with commitment to follow-up care can be assured of infection prevention.

What are the risks of antibiotic treatment in the eyes?

- RISK OF ANTIBIOTIC RESISTANCE: There are several ways that bacteria develop antibiotic resistance, including overuse of antibiotics in the hospital, community, and farms; use of low doses over long periods of time; and high levels of resistant bacteria being present (there is power in numbers!). If a child develops a resistance to certain

292 The Essential Homebirth Guide

antibiotics and becomes ill, they will require ever-stronger medication to fight infection.

- PAIN FOR THE NEWBORN: The possible side effects associated with the medicine include some stinging, irritation, itching, redness, blurred vision (lasting about thirty minutes), and sensitivity to light.[11]

- BLURRED VISION FOR THE NEWBORN: This is one of the potential side effects listed by the manufacturer. Your baby's vision capabilities at birth allow for a particular interaction with you. Interrupting this disrupts the bonding process.[12]

- POTENTIAL TO MISS AN INFECTION PRESENT IN THE MOTHER: If a mother carries gonococcal bacteria but has no symptoms, as is the case in around 80 percent of infected women, and the baby is treated preemptively, colonization of the gonococcal bacteria can grow unchecked on the mother. This results in pelvic inflammatory disease (PID). PID can lead to internal abscesses (pus-filled "pockets" that are hard to cure) and long-lasting, chronic pelvic pain. PID can damage the fallopian tubes enough to cause infertility or increase the risk of a future ectopic pregnancy.[13]

To Treat or Not to Treat: Is my baby at risk for this infection?

IF YOU DO NOT know or trust your partner's sexual history, this treatment is the first level available to directly prevent the transmission of gonorrhea from you to your baby. A less-direct approach would be to carefully watch your baby for development of an eye infection and then seek appropriate medical care.

The complications from a newborn eye infection from gonorrhea are severe, appear rapidly, and are likely to cause blindness if left untreated. The transmission rate for gonorrhea from an infected mother to her baby is 30 to 50 percent.[14]

I have decided to have my baby treated; how is the ointment applied?

A LINE OF OINTMENT 1 to 2 centimeters long is placed in the lower eye. The closed eyelids may be gently massaged to help spread the solution. After one minute, any excess ointment is gently wiped from the eyelids and surrounding skin with sterile cotton. The eyes should not be irrigated in any way after the ointment is put in or the effectiveness may be compromised.[15] Ideally, you will hold your baby while the medication is given.

I feel very confident about my and my partner's sexual history. I want to opt out of this treatment.

THIS IS A VALID choice for many families. We have seen a lot more parents refuse this medication than accept it. In many states, your midwife will require you to sign a form stating that you have refused treatment.

We trust most homebirth families are aware and watchful during the postpartum time. Babies with eye infections have goopy red eyes that get crusted over. If you notice these symptoms in your newborn, call your midwife or pediatrician right away.

What is Newborn Screening, and will my midwife perform this?

NEWBORN SCREENING IS A process that screens your baby for multiple endocrine, metabolic, and genetic disorders at one time. It is done by pricking your baby's foot and collecting a blood sample on a special card. This card is then sent to a laboratory and if any of the screens are positive, the family is notified and further diagnostic testing is offered.

Some midwives will ask to do a screen during the immediate hours following birth, and then perform a second check at the first postpartum office visit. This visit usually takes place between one and two weeks after the birth. Some midwives skip the first screen, and only do the second.

Which disorders are being screened for?

THIS VARIES FROM STATE to state. PKU (a genetic disorder), cystic fibrosis, and sickle-cell anemia are found on most states' screens. For more specific information, contact your state's Department of Health.

Are there any risks to the screen?

THERE IS OF COURSE some pain involved in any blood collection, and there is always a slight risk of infection at the collection site.

What are the benefits of the screen?

MANY OF THESE DISEASES are treatable if caught early. It is not always possible to know if a baby has one of these disorders just by looking or through a routine physical. Newborn Screening is a tool that can help identify children with these disorders so that treatment can begin as soon as possible.

Postpartum Depression

What is postpartum depression?

POSTPARTUM DEPRESSION (PPD) SEEMS like a contradiction. You've just had a baby. You're supposed to be on top of the world. Sure, you expected the exhaustion, and were prepared for your life to be reorganized in a way that might take some getting used to, but this is something completely different.

Many women, up to 85 percent, experience minor fluctuations in mood after birth, which can persist up to two weeks postpartum.[16] This is known as the baby blues, and is a normal part of the hormonal shift your body makes as it goes from being pregnant to not pregnant.

Postpartum depression makes you doubt your entire self and your decision to share your life with your baby. You may feel anxious, lose what little sleep you might get, and have scary repetitive thoughts. You may not be able to properly care for your baby. It can be debilitating and frightening, and when you are in the thick of it, can be almost completely overwhelming.

How common is postpartum depression?

IT'S MORE COMMON THAN you might think. Studies have shown that up to 15 percent of all mothers are diagnosed with PPD sometime during the first year of their child's life.[17] The American Congress of Obstetricians and Gynecologists recommends that all women be screened for PPD between four and six weeks postpartum. The midwifery Model of Care provides between four and six visits within the first six weeks postpartum. This allows for earlier and more consistent opportunities for screening and early treatment.

Am I at risk for postpartum depression?

ONE OF THE BIGGEST risk factors for PPD is a history of depression. If you have been depressed before, regardless of the trigger, you have a 30 to 62 percent chance of experiencing a postpartum mood disorder.[18] Other risk factors include

1. inadequate support, especially from your partner and/or family

2. financial difficulties

3. unplanned pregnancy

4. teenage pregnancy

5. single parenting

6. family history of depression

7. history of sexual abuse

8. a traumatic birth experience

I believe I am at risk. What can I do?

IDEALLY, IF YOU HAVE risk factors (and even if you don't), it's a great idea to chat with your midwife prenatally about the possibility of PPD. If you have a history of depression, share what treatments have worked for you in the past. If you know you need more support at home, your midwife can help you locate a postpartum doula. These professionals specialize in helping new parents adjust to their new life and can do everything from providing a listening ear to doing your laundry and dishes. They can help with basic breastfeeding issues, entertain your older children, and take your dog for a walk. They are especially helpful when you do not have family locally.

It is extremely important that you take good care of yourself during this period. Now, that may look completely different than it did prebaby. It is important to get as much sleep as you can, nourish your body with nutrient-dense food, and surround yourself with people and things that uplift you.

The best midwives are those who will help you see your postpartum time in a realistic light, especially for you first timers. Keep your expectations low and reasonable. Your house will not be perfectly clean. You may skip a shower or two. Your other children may be wearing some interesting outfits. This is okay! In fact, it shows us that you are doing everything right. The first few weeks are a transitional time, where you should be doing nothing but caring for your baby and yourself. There is so much value in this, yet our society does not recognize it. In fact, it glorifies the opposite. It may seem as if you are expected to have everything under control three days after birth. If you feel like you have to be Superwoman, you are just setting yourself up for failure, which has tipped many women over the edge.

Is this treatable, or do I just have to tough it out?

GOOD NEWS! PPD IS a very treatable illness. For many years, health care providers thought that PPD was its own disease, completely separate from other forms of depression. Now we know that while the cause may be different, the brain reacts very similarly, from a chemical standpoint, in all forms of depressive illness. This is such a positive discovery. Any treatment that has worked for depression is on the table for PPD. This can range from traditional talk therapy all the way up to psychotropic medications. You have many options.

Can I do anything else to decrease my risks?

YOU ARE ALREADY DOING it, or at least thinking about it. Having a homebirth can make a big difference in your mood during this time. The medical world has some good research showing that the more informed patients are, and the more control they have over their experience, the less likely they are to become depressed during their recovery.[19] There is nowhere that you will feel more in control than in your own home. Your house is your refuge and your castle, and midwives are very aware that they are invited guests.

It has been known for some time that midwifery care itself decreases PPD.[20] (Interestingly, this study does not differentiate between homebirth midwives and hospital midwives. It was conducted in the UK, where midwives are expected to be proficient in both types of care.) Like everything else addressed in this book, it goes back to respect and relationships. Midwifery care is 90 percent listening, 10 percent doing, and 100 percent about the relationship. Women are not meant to go through their pregnancy, birth, and recovery alone. It is not optimum from any standpoint, biological or psychological. You need accurate knowledge, loving support, and respect for your ideas and intuition. Sounds like midwifery care!

In a Web-published study, Michelle Bland of Missouri Western State University gives scientific credence to the intuitive feeling that homebirth is a great choice for those prone to PPD. She compared the rates of depression in mothers who birthed at home and those who birthed in the hospital. She further differentiated between mothers who birthed vaginally in the hospital and those who had cesarean sections. She found PPD rates are lowest among homebirthers.[21]

Amanda's experience backs this up.

> With my first child, I didn't know what to expect so I just went with the hospital. My labor started with my water breaking, and they were not satisfied with my progress, so they gave me Pitocin. This was extremely intense, although I did manage without any pain medication. Although I was in labor for twenty hours, I only pushed for thirty minutes; I tore badly, and the repair was worse than labor! They took my daughter away while they were doing this and I just wanted to nurse her. I remember being happy and in love when she was born, although looking back, I can see that the bonding with her was a little different than with my two other children. My recovery was long and my bottom was swollen for a long time. I kept thinking, "I don't want to do this again anytime soon." I developed thrush, and for almost *two years* after the birth I suffered from postpartum depression. I wanted more kids but I didn't think I would be able to because of how terrible I felt. I just could not imagine going through this again.
>
> I have a four-and-one-half year gap between my first and second children. I was that scared of postpartum depression. With my second child, I did a lot of reading and talking to friends who had homebirths and thought this sounded like a good fit for me. I prepared as much as I could for the postpartum depression to happen again. I had my second daughter at home in the middle of the night. It was a peaceful and fast labor. She was born four hours after my water broke and it took only three pushes kneeling at the side of my bed to birth this little girl. My midwife barely made it!
>
> The first thing I thought when I saw her was "I love you so much!" The second was, "I want to have another baby at home." She was such a sweet little spirit. No one took her from

my arms. I was triumphant, happy, joyful, and full of energy. She nursed right away with no problem and I helped wipe her off a little with a warm washcloth. I got to hold her for a good hour before they needed to take her and do the newborn stuff, but she was right next to me the whole time. I did not tear and my recovery was faster and easier this time. For days and weeks, I would daydream while nursing about how wonderful and perfect the birth was, and how I couldn't wait to do it again. It was so much different than how I felt after my first. I did not have any postpartum depression. At all! I couldn't believe it! I felt so good, we planned the third baby soon after.

My third baby was a boy born at home two years later. He had a very different delivery. He came at night during a snowstorm and a full moon, and we were worried that our midwife would not be able to get to us, due to the weather. She did, though! Labor was about four hours long. The pushing was harder than my first two. When his head finally came out, I pushed, but his body would not move. I was on my knees again and heard the urgency in my midwife's voice when she told me to flip over so she could help me better. I pushed really hard again, the midwife turned him, and he finally came out. I remember feeling such relief, but my son did not breathe right away and was blue. I held him, talked to him, and rubbed his back and he slowly started taking breaths. It was so amazing. I felt instant love, joy, and peace, just like with my second baby. We bonded easily in those postbirth moments. Again, there was no tearing, even with all the drama down there. I did keep thinking how much harder it was to push this baby out than with my second. I felt very triumphant. And you know what? Even with a birth experience that could have been perceived as stressful, I still did not have postpartum depression!

—Amanda

Sometimes, however, PPD just happens. There can be no risk factors at all, and you can have the most beautiful homebirth, and still experience PPD. Liz's experience reflects this:

I had my fourth child, a daughter, in the tub in my bathroom, almost twelve years ago. I woke up in labor, had breakfast, birthed her at lunchtime, and had dinner with the family in the evening. All rather smooth. Too smooth, really. Her birth was idyllic by all normal birth measures. She was perfect. It was fabulous to not drive anywhere in labor, and it was lovely to rest in my own bed afterward. My midwife made me scrambled eggs, which I ate in bed. Delicious.

Unlike her brothers' births (two hospital, one birth center), I felt no flicker of joy. I pretended. The photos looked joyful, but I was feeling empty. The flow of the day left it all feeling rather anticlimactic. I missed the ritual of "bringing the baby home."

My daughter wasn't a particularly attractive newborn—all smooshy with way too much dark hair to be one of "my" babies. She went on to develop colic and was a demanding baby and toddler. She was also one child too many for my ability to cope (she was a surprise from the start!). In retrospect, it was all a great setup for postpartum depression, which I finally acknowledged when she was six months old.

My biggest regret is that at my final postpartum visit with my midwife, when she asked "How's everything going?" I responded with what I felt was the ideal answer, "Oh, yes! Everything's great!" But the truth (which I hadn't even faced myself) was I was merely surviving.

I wanted to share this because homebirth is no vaccination against mood disorders. If I had a fifth baby, I would for sure plan a homebirth. But I would be much more careful to critique my well-being afterward. I would also make sure that my loved ones knew to really question how well I was doing. And I would plan a ritual to welcome the baby.

—Liz

Postpartum depression is not a normal part of having a baby. It is a serious illness, which can be treated. We encourage you to seek help as soon as you or your loved ones realize something is not quite right. One excellent resource is Postpartum Support International, a worldwide organization dedicated to helping women with postpartum mood disorders. You can find them on the Web at www.postpartum .net. Remember that you are not alone and there is help.

What kind of follow-up care should I expect?

YOUR MIDWIFE WILL VISIT you at home in the first week after birth, and you will receive follow-up care for yourself and your baby for at least six weeks postpartum. This care is designed to ensure that your baby is thriving and that you are healing well. It provides opportunities to reflect upon your birth story, celebrate your success, and gain understanding around anything that you cannot make sense of. You can ask your midwife questions about breastfeeding and newborn care, as well as discuss the changes to your body as you move further away from pregnancy. At the final visit, your midwife will help you with family planning and offer you a PAP smear.

Most families and midwives feel a sense of sadness at that last appointment. The relationship between a woman and her midwife is sacred and unique. Stay in touch with her—we haven't met a midwife who does not love receiving pictures on birthdays or notes from time to time. The relationship you developed with your midwife may be part and parcel of midwifery work, but just like it nurtured you, it has great meaning to her, as well.

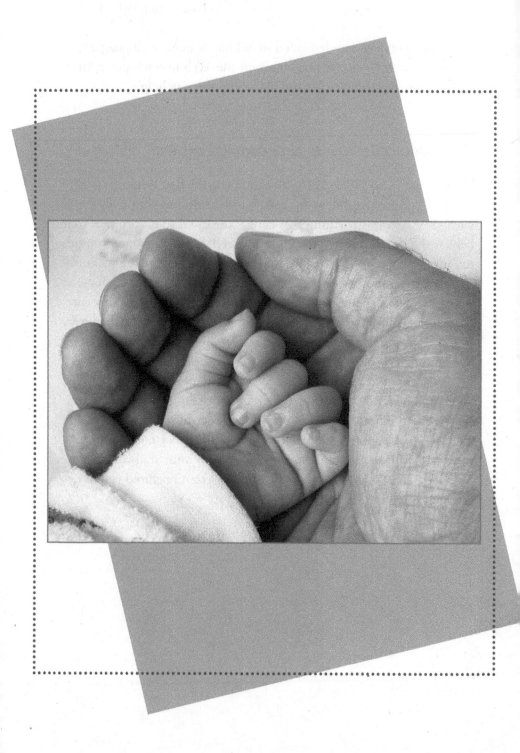

CHAPTER TWELVE

The Story Continues

MAMA SAYS

For the first time, I truly understand the meaning of the words "unconditional love." I am so deeply in love, with my experience, and with my family, that it would be impossible for me to ever dig my way out. It is a good thing I'd never want to.

—Sasha

WE STARTED WITH "ONCE upon a time," so what's the logical ending? "And they lived happily ever after," of course! But the story doesn't end there. It never does. Birth of all kinds, of a baby, of a book, of a nation, is always just the beginning. As wonderful as it is, home-birth is merely the starting point for the rest of your life, one that now includes a brand new human being. To birth the next generation from and into an environment of health is so big. It is impossible to experience something so profound and not come away changed.

This is true empowerment. Homebirthing forces you to dig deep, to create your reality in ways that run contrary to the mainstream, knowing it is your truth. It makes you evaluate and re-evaluate your values, and gives you the unique opportunity to actually live your aspirations. This gentle, wild, awesome way of birthing is rooted in the very oldest of human needs: connection and love. In homebirthing you can't have one without the other; they spill and splash all over everyone involved and nobody is ever quite the same.

In this spirit of community and tenderness, we want to gift you with some inspiration. The stories that follow are from your sisters, your mothers, and your friends. They come from all over the country and from all different kinds of families. They are you, and you are they. You have faced the same fears, the same questions, and have all found value in birthing normally and intentionally. Welcome home.

Bethany's Story

ABOUT FOUR DAYS PAST Elsa's due date, after dealing with bed rest for preterm labor from 24 weeks on, she finally decided to come! I had been about 2 or 3 centimeters dilated and 75 percent effaced for a couple of weeks. I had never dilated or progressed before labor in any way with my other two kids. We were sure Elsa would come quite early, at least as soon as I was off bed rest at 37 weeks. I began to get very discouraged about the time of her due date, believing that maybe I had so succeeded in stopping labor that it would never begin on its own.

My midwife assured me that it would, but I don't think I believed her. I was pleased, though, that at each appointment I had progressed just a little more than the week before. I told Dennis, my husband, several times, that if I could just continue to progress without painful contractions, maybe I wouldn't begin active labor until I was significantly dilated. Then maybe my labor would be very short! I was really encouraged by that thought. The last couple of weeks, each time I would feel a contraction, I would move my hips and think downward thoughts, just to see how much progression I could get out of each contraction.

The day before labor began, I e-mailed the midwife saying that I was really discouraged, had had no signs of labor at all that day, and was just done. Dennis told me that it was just the calm before the storm. I went to bed resigned to the idea of never giving birth to this stubborn baby.

I couldn't sleep. About one thirty in the morning I began to get sharp pains in my pubic area. I was moaning and squirming around, trying to make it stop. I got onto all fours, did pelvic rocking, and eventually could only find relief in a knee-chest position. I couldn't watch the clock to see if any of the pain could be timed because it was too intense and almost nonstop. I could feel the baby making huge movements in the pelvis that triggered the pain. Finally, at 2:45, the movement and pain stopped and I fell asleep.

I awoke again at 4:00 a.m. to a painful contraction! This was something fairly new, and I knew I would be giving birth that day. It occurred to me then that the hour of movement I had experienced earlier was the baby moving herself into the perfect position for birth. The contractions continued for a full hour, five to ten minutes apart. I laid on my left side and relaxed and breathed deeply through each one. I finally couldn't tolerate them laying down and got up at five to pace through them. I didn't stop walking for almost an hour, even during contractions.

They began to hurt worse and were consistently less than seven minutes apart, so I e-mailed my doula to tell her I would be calling later in the day and woke up Dennis. I told him it was time to start filling the tub! The contractions got progressively longer, stronger and closer together, so Dennis called my doula and asked her to come. We called the midwife at eight in the morning. The birth assistant told us that the midwife was occupied but could plan to be to us in a few hours.

I decided not to worry and to take a nap. I slept in twenty to thirty-minute segments in between average-strength contractions. I got up at ten thirty-ish, around the time my doula arrived. My contractions had slowed way down at this point. We talked and I showed her all of my birth gear. She then asked when exactly labor had slowed. I mentioned that it was when the kids woke up. She suggested seeing what would happen if they left, so my mom came and took them.

Slowly but surely the contractions returned. They got more and more painful until they were lasting sixty to ninety seconds each and were six to seven minutes apart. By one thirty in the afternoon, the pain dramatically increased and we called the midwife again. She asked to speak to me and I told her things were moving fast. Immediately after hanging up with her, I moved to lean over my birth ball and the contractions became two to three minutes apart, lasting almost as long. I still didn't want anyone talking or touching me during them. I remember saying then that I was scared it would never end and I couldn't take much more of this. I tried to stand up but was shaking. I recognized transition. So did the doula and Dennis. They immediately called the midwife back and told her to hurry. The midwives were just leaving their birth center and would be there in thirty to forty minutes. No one knew if I'd make it that long.

As the contractions came back to back, I knew this was my chance to get in the tub. I went into my room, chose the candle scent I wanted, picked out a CD to play, and crawled in. The tub was 104 degrees, too hot. So I asked for ice to be dumped in.

I desperately wanted to stay in the tub, but had to use the potty. As each incredibly painful contraction came, I cried out and my doula would come to push on my back and encourage me. I was so demanding, crying, "Harder! No! Stop! Again! Push!" It occurred to me several times that my doula was pregnant also and I was expecting an awful lot out of her, but I couldn't seem to cope without her help.

As I stood over the toilet, not able to decide if I should attempt to go back to the tub, my doula announced with relief, "They're here!"

The midwife later told Dennis that they had arrived in only twenty-nine minutes! A record! I tried to walk the ten steps to the tub but only made it two steps. I tried to whisper-communicate that I couldn't get in the tub, because I'd just have to get back out again, but I couldn't tell if anyone could understand me. The birth assistant ushered me to the tub as I clung to her, hardly able to move. Eventually she was able to nearly lift me into it. She gave me a stool to put my left foot on to relieve the intense pain in my left hip.

The midwife asked if I wanted to try pushing or get checked first. Definitely get checked. She said, "Oh! The head is right there, only this far in." And she showed me a couple of inches with her fingers. It still didn't register with me that I was completely dilated, until my doula said, "You were hoping for six centimeters and you're complete!" My midwife asked when my water had broken. I had completely forgotten about it! I didn't know.

I asked if I could push and they said of course. It didn't feel like a relief at all to push this time, unlike my other births. It felt like hard, unnatural work and I hated it. But I hated being in labor more, so I pushed. I could feel nothing happening. I decided to see for myself if the baby was even near coming out. I reached in and could feel her head just a couple of inches inside! I announced that I felt her! Yes! I was pumped! This was my first homebirth after two hospital births, and I had really wanted to be aware and alert at this birth. I had always felt in the past that I was out of control, and that the birth "happened" to me instead of my making the birth happen.

I was leaning over the side of the tub, biting the edge, and then resting my face against it. I was ready to push her out. I gave a couple of tiny pushes, then at once realized the baby was filling the vaginal canal: a totally new sensation—not painful at all, just different. I announced that she was coming! I slowly, barely pushed and felt her crown. I figured she was at least 9 pounds, so as she crowned, I waited, letting her stretch me. As I simply waited with her at the opening, I didn't feel burning or stretching pain, just her head, right there.

My midwife said to very slowly push, so I just barely did. She supported the perineum and said that I was going very slowly, just right. I didn't feel an urge to push, so it was easy to not go fast! I was told that part of her head was out and I needed to push the rest out. I didn't want to. I didn't understand why no one could just pull her out. I ignored them all and waited for (Dennis told me later) about two minutes to give another push. Then I felt the rest of her body slowly come out of me. I heard the midwife announce "tight cord" as I turned over to sit on a stool in the tub. She worked to unwrap the cord from around Elsa's neck and then I was handed my baby!

Beautiful, pink, tiny little Elsa! She cried and looked right into my eyes! I couldn't stop crying! I had done it! I had given birth, in the water, to my perfect little girl! One of the most joyful moments of my life!

Colleen's Story

MY BABY JOSEPH WAS born at home. I just want to shout that so you all can hear it. He was born at home! AT HOME!

I had nine days of irregular contractions. Each day they grew a little stronger and lasted longer. By day nine they were coming every ten minutes all day long. My husband, Jimmie, stayed up with me that night and we kept track until four in the morning. I finally fell asleep.

I woke up at eight thirty. The morning went by with contractions every three to twenty minutes. They grew stronger. My doula showed up around noon. When I awoke from trying to nap for a few hours, labor picked up rapidly. Within the next hour they were consistently every four minutes or so. This was around four. By five in the evening, my doula and my mom agreed to call my midwife.

When she and her assistant arrived, I was kneeling and holding on to the back of the couch with my head pressing into the wall. I was already wondering how I was going to keep going. It hurt! I was not expecting that much pain. How much longer might it be? Soon I was checked and was 7 centimeters. That sounds good, but it wasn't good enough for me! Then I remembered the candles from my mama blessing. My husband lit them, but by that time, I was too deep into labor to think about the positive affirmations and energy they represented. I was deep, deep, deep.

I was in my bedroom the whole time the candles were burning and then my midwife suggested I walk. So I held on to her and my doula and walked to the front room. The contractions were two minutes apart and I was bending over in pain and moaning. I went back to the couch and felt like I could just not go on. Three women around me were telling me, "Colleen, you can do it! Focus on your baby and not the pain."

I was saying, "No! I can't handle the pain anymore. I need a shot or an epidural. This is unbearable!" My midwife reminded me that the mind is very powerful. I tried to think about the cervix opening and let the pain move through me. But soon I was saying that I wanted to go to the hospital *now*. My team completely respected me, and we got ready to go to the hospital.

I was standing by the front door with my husband while everyone else was preparing to leave, and I told him I was going to go pee before we left. No more than two minutes later, I was sitting on the toilet, my mucous plug came out, and I began to push involuntarily.

I knew I was not leaving home at that point. I was going to have my baby at home whether I believed I could deal with the pain or not. So, okay.

When my midwife came back inside from her car, I asked, "Is there *anything* we can do to make this more bearable?" It turned out the assistant had a birthing tub in her trunk. It was set up in no time in my front room. While it was being filled, I was standing and hanging on to Jimmie and my doula, moaning loudly with each contraction. As soon as it was filled, I got in. I knelt against the edge of the tub; it was a good position to be in for pushing. The water felt good. Jimmie got in soon after me and applied pressure to my hips during my contractions and it really helped, too. I think I was only in the tub for about fifteen minutes before my baby was born, with one last big push. I am a great pusher!

Joseph was lifted gently onto my chest with the cord still pulsing. I was kind of in shock. I just had a baby at home in my front room in a birthing tub! I couldn't believe it. The homebirth was planned. The waterbirth was something that happened in the last hour. It was great.

Afterward I was physically exhausted, but I was on a high from the birth that prevented me from going right to sleep. I lay awake in my bed for hours with the new baby just stroking hair, smelling skin, eating, and breastfeeding. When we all finally went to sleep, I got to sleep for four hours straight. What I really liked was being able to nurse my baby when he was hungry, not according to a nurse's schedule like I had to in the hospital. They would not have let me go for so long without waking me and my baby to nurse. But at home we nursed when Baby wanted and that worked perfectly.

I believed in myself for the entire pregnancy. I purposely did not tell many people that we were planning a homebirth because I wanted to keep away doubts and negativity. Then in labor, I was fine until the last few hours. That is when I didn't believe I could do it anymore. The midwives, my doula, my mom, and Jimmie all believed I could, though. With their support, I was able to deliver Joseph at home, and doing that transformed me. I am a woman who now knows she is much stronger than she thought. This was the hardest thing I have ever done, but I feel so proud of myself and truly thankful for such an experience.

Robbi's Story

MY STORY STARTS BEFORE my first daughter was born over four and one half years ago. I did my research before I got pregnant and found a midwife and birth center that would take my insurance. I had always thought if everything goes right and well at the birth center, I could definitely imagine having the rest of my babies at home. I knew I wanted something different from the hospital; I wanted a natural birth with a midwife.

My first two babies were both very malpositioned and the labors were both very long and led to cesareans. When I became pregnant again, I knew in my heart that I could not just schedule another c-section. I had to try to birth this last baby vaginally. There was just something so missing in my life as a mother. It just tore me up inside. Luckily I knew a wonderful midwife who was willing to help me try for a homebirth.

My labor began early in the morning. I woke up with labor pains, and labored on my own in my living room and kitchen area while my family slept. I focused on myself and my baby through the dark night and early morning. I remember calling my midwife around 2:00 a.m. to give her the heads-up.

I was three hours into labor and this was my first baby out of three that wasn't giving me terrible back pain. I *loved* not having to have an IV or being poked and prodded. I started feeling a little pushy around 5:30.

I was happy to feel that pressure sensation and pushiness that I had not felt in my prior labors. It was about 8:40 a.m. when I was in the water and my body was pushing a little on its own with each contraction . . . what an amazing feeling! Could I really be at 10 centimeters already? I just couldn't believe it, as my other labors had been so long. I told my husband to call my midwife again; what if she didn't make it? I can't even describe the relief I felt when she walked in, along with her assistant and my doula. I felt awesome, so supported, and to top it all off, it was a beautiful summer morning.

Because they were with me, I felt I could really just let my body push. I got out of the tub and went to the toilet to pee, and pushed a bit there. I had my first check (at my request) nearly nine hours into labor. I think the sweetest words I had ever heard were, "Oh, hi Baby! Robbi, you're completely dilated, and the head is right there."

It's funny: for four and a half years I had always imagined this beautiful birth taking place in the water but the bed is where I ended up. I had actually asked for a catheter because I could not pee for the life of me, and that is where I stayed. It was totally fine.

I pushed hard and my midwife helped get the baby's shoulder out because it was stuck. I feel I gave birth for the first time, even though it was my third baby, that summer morning. I was surrounded by skilled support and just felt so loved. Three wonderful ladies held me and took pictures, and my husband was absolutely amazing. My four and a half year old and my two year old got to meet their new sister right away. To this day, when my oldest talks about the birth, she says to me, "Mommy, I'm glad you gave birth so well!"

Sometimes I get teary eyed because I wasn't able to give "birth *well"* to my first two babies. My daughter used to think that babies came out of a line in my stomach, but now she really knows where babies come from and she isn't afraid.

Giving birth to my baby in my home with so much support has resolved *a lot* of emotional angst in my life. For almost five years I have obsessed over what had gone wrong, what I could have done differently. I was so grief ridden that it was making me bitter. Then, in one eleven-hour period, these feelings nearly disappeared. I finally feel like a "mother," a "woman," a "wife." I now feel like the incredibly hard work I put into trying to have my first two babies was for a reason. It was not a complete waste of time. It led me to this moment, and all I want is for other mothers to get to feel like I do now.

April's Story

OUR BABY'S DUE DATE was March 2 but she was born on March 17, so this made her entrance into the world fifteen days "late." Those were the hardest days! It was like anticipating a bomb could go off at any moment. As the clocked ticked down, so did my option of a birth center birth since they only allow mothers to deliver there between 37 and 42 weeks.

My midwives kept reminding me that I always had the option for a homebirth. As we got further away from the due date, I accepted the fact that I might be doing this at home.

On Wednesday, March 16, I woke up and realized that I had lost my mucus plug. Lots of mucus kind of gushed out. I informed my midwives and doula and they told me to go about my day, as it could be a while before anything happens.

So that's what I did. I ate breakfast, went for a morning walk, and then later met up with my brother and went to a lake near our house. All in all, it was a nice day.

At two thirty the next morning, I woke up with a contraction that startled me. It felt really strong. I went to the bathroom and saw more blood-streaked mucus like the day before. I started to go back to bed but then about five minutes later, another strong contraction came. I timed them for the next hour. They were consistently over one minute long and about five minutes apart. At three thirty I woke up my husband because they were just so painful. The contractions were closer together and lasting longer. This time they were so painful that I was shaking. I was thinking, "This is happening way too fast! Where was all my prelabor stuff?" My contractions went from nothing to hard labor faster than a Maserati.

We called the midwives and my doula and they listened to me through contractions. My midwife said, "I'm coming to your house right now." She said it with a bit of urgency, but I didn't know what to make of it.

Around four forty-five I felt like I needed to push. The midwives and doula had not arrived yet. I said, "Call them!!!" He did and they were ten minutes away. She told me to breathe through the contractions.

As soon as the team got to our apartment, my midwife checked me and said, "Well, you are at nine centimeters. Don't push yet." At that point it was also decided that we wouldn't even try to get to the birth center, which was a twenty-minute car ride away. I didn't want to get in a car and I was way far along in my labor. There was a part of me that didn't care about *where* I had the baby, I was more concerned with *how* I was going to have the baby. I do recall feeling amazed that my body had dilated so fast.

I felt I had to push a little with each contraction. Not with all my might, but slowly at the peak of each contraction. I changed positions to help cope with immense pressure I was feeling. I especially liked sitting backward on the toilet, and squatting while holding on to the bed. I kept telling my team, "I need to poop, but nothing will come out." After a lot of pushing, my midwife had me try new positions to help my baby out. It felt like it was taking a long time and I kept watching the clock. At some point my husband realized this and took it off the wall so that I wouldn't worry.

I felt the baby move a lot and the pushing was very intense. It was the whole stretching of everything. It felt like it was burning. When her head started to come through, it was an intense burning sensation! Ring of fire! They had me slow down so I could stretch. Then they realized she had a hand up, which is why the pushing was so long. She was moving through with an arm up right at her chin. One of the midwives helped move her arm down so the rest of the head could come.

I birthed her head with short grunting pushes. I felt her head with my hand—it was amazing! They told me to give one big push with the next contraction. I pushed her whole body out and my husband Sean caught her. She was wide awake and resting on my chest. She was coughing and breathing but not really crying. Her eyes were wide and she was looking around. When Sean talked to her, she looked right at him.

We spent the next three hours cuddling in bed, getting cleaned up, and eating a delicious meal one of the midwives made for us. Our team let us enjoy and be with each other. They didn't rush to do anything or interrupt us from getting to know each other.

Having the homebirth experience was amazing. I felt empowered. It was cozy. I still vividly remember the feeling of putting on my pajamas, snuggling up in bed, and holding my daughter. It was amazing to never leave home. She was born into an environment that we felt safe in. There wasn't any trauma or whisking her away. It was us, just us, in our own world.

My experience was amazing! I never once wanted to go to the hospital. Even though in the heat of transition I yelled something about any woman who gives birth being crazy, my whole experience was just fantastic.

Sasha's Story

MY FIRST DAUGHTER'S BIRTH was by far the most painful (yet amazing!) experience of my entire life on this earth. After nineteen hours of labor, nine with excruciating back pain, I felt like an absolute warrior for months following. I felt like I could conquer the world.

I had thought I could do it, have a natural birth at home, but to actually accomplish it was a whole different thing. The power it gives you as a human being is absolutely undeniable; it completely changed me as a person. I've been a registered nurse in the postpartum department at a very mainstream hospital for almost eight years. Having my own children, and experiencing midwifery care and homebirth, has completely changed the way I practice.

It actually was incredibly difficult to go back into the hospital setting after having my first baby. I see nothing but intervention there, some good, but honestly, mostly bad. It is so hard to teach philosophies that I don't necessarily believe in as an individual and as a woman. I often have to bite my tongue and refrain from giving my opinion. I often wonder if I'll be able to continue working in a setting where intervention is so highly regarded and a more natural approach is so frowned upon.

I have since inspired a few friends of mine to use a homebirth midwife, all with successful births and beautiful memories. Now that I've experienced two homebirths and two painful back labors, many people in my life regard me as a Superwoman. While I do feel wonderful about my homebirth experiences, I know that anyone is capable of what I have done. You just have to want it, and believe in yourself. You must turn within yourself to find the strength. Homebirth has made me a stronger and more confident woman. It has definitely made me a better person, a better mother, and a better nurse.

Penny's Story

I UNDERSTAND THAT MANY VBAC mamas have some fears about laboring and getting to or past the point where things went wrong in the birth of their child that led to their c-section. I'm no different, but I never labored with my son at all. Placenta previa was the culprit for our c-section birth, so laboring wasn't allowed. For us, the biggest fear was prematurity, since Gavin was ripped from my body, I mean *born*, at 33½ weeks. He had to be on a ventilator, then CPAP, then ventilator again, under the lights for jaundice, etc. . . . He had so many interventions, and a hospital staff that took over his care and kept us on their schedules and rules. So, naturally, we were terrified of a do-over of that experience. I was really anxious and jumpy any time I got overtired and my Braxton Hicks got out of control. Not until I hit week 34 did I really breathe easy and let go of the potential for this pregnancy to be another extended traumatic experience.

On the day of the birth . . .

I get up early in the morning to feed the cat and use the bathroom. I am so excited to see bloody show! Well, I have plenty of time; this is sure to take around twenty-four hours once contractions start. I'll just go back to our birth books and mark the important parts. *The Birth Partner*, done. *The Pregnancy Book*, done. *The Bradley Method*, done. *Natural Childbirth the Bradley Way*, done. Now I'm refreshed on the emotional signposts. I'm set. Several more trips to the toilet and lots more bloody show, cool. Okay, now get some rest while you can! But take an apple with you. Yeah, an apple is a good idea, and a Baker's Breakfast cookie, yum-yum.

I rest and wait. And wait. Then, I feel what I now think of as a dilating contraction. I've worked out that I'll use the mantra from one of Ina May Gaskin's birth stories, "I'm getting HUGE," to welcome contractions. I can't wait!

We'd bought a neat gadget called Labor'Lert a couple weeks before to time contractions. Push the button at the beginning and end of each contraction, and it keeps track of how long they last and intervals between. Roger's job is to keep track of the contractions, and we decide for me to just yell "Push it!" at the beginning and end of contractions. Okay, I missed that first one. Let's get the next for sure. At 5:33 in the morning, I get my chance. They are seventeen minutes apart. Hmmm. This is going to be a long day; she might not get here until tomorrow. At 5:42, another one hits. Oh, already getting closer together. Good, maybe today. Too soon to know what might change. This could all stop, especially if I can get to sleep. We time another couple, then try to sleep to see if they stop. 5:50 a.m. 5:57 a.m. Uh-huh, this is picking up! So much for sleep. Put the machine down and close your eyes! Rest, contraction, rest, contraction.

At 6:15, I wake Roger up and get him to fill the tub. I also want to get one last photo of my pregnant belly before it's gone. I know that this is crazy, but it's important to me. I get dressed in my special photo outfit and we get the shot. By this time the contractions are about three and a half minutes apart, so we call our doula, who is also our midwife's assistant. She has an hour-long drive to get to us, and rush hour is starting, so we want to give her the heads-up.

By 7:45, I'm in the bathroom trying to poop again. Now, alone in the bathroom, while Roger deals with Gavin throwing a screwdriver, I think that I could go to the hospital and have this done inside of two hours. Not how I planned, but . . . Then I glimpse myself in the mirror, and give myself a good scolding. "Shut up, you can do this! Don't forget they almost killed you with a *necessary* cesarean; don't give them the chance with an *un*necessary one!" Enter Roger with, "Tub's ready when you are." Hallelujah!

At 9:07 a.m. we call our midwife. We need to slow this down, this is too intense, and we want some professional direction. Yep, I'll go ahead and get in the tub now. At least it will ease some of the intensity of these contractions! Roger speaks to the midwife, tells her the contractions are about two minutes apart and lasting one and a half minutes.

At 9:40 a.m. our doula arrives. Happy day! We are definitely having a baby. I eat some eggs. They are kind of gross, but I choke them down. I head back into the bathroom, as I feel I have to poop with every contraction. It hurts a lot to sit there, but somehow, I can't seem to move.

At 10:40 the doula senses something I don't and asks, "Do you want to push?" Oh, my gosh, with that question, I suddenly realize and tell her, "*Yes*, I'm going to push *right now!* But can I get back in the tub?" She nods yes and I get in.

Our doula says something about trying to breathe through the contractions if I can, but to do what my body is telling me to do. I don't actually want to, but I just can't help it. Roger gets in the tub with me and pushes on my back. I lean back into him. Push, Push, Push.

I'm holding my perineum, and feel my bag of waters in my vagina. It's so cool! Next push, the bag of waters is a little balloon outside my body. Another push. Resting, bag of waters breaks. Push, crowning— wow, that burns, but then she goes back in a bit. Push, out she comes a little bit more. I ask, "Is that her head? It's all wrinkly!" Push, more burning, let's stop for a few minutes. I wish I could, but my body is just doing its thing without me!

The midwife isn't here, yet. She calls on the doula's phone. Our doula is giving directions, then puts the phone on speaker. I'm still pushing. Roger and I join in: "Turn around. Past McDonald's, turn right. It's a light, turn right at the light at 7-Eleven. Watch for a bunch of garbage cans, then turn just past those into the driveway." Push, her head is out! The cord is around her neck. And our doula puts on her midwife's assistant hat and gently says, "Breathe through while I get the cord unwrapped." Just then, the midwife flies into the house, adrenaline pumping. She takes over and unwraps the cord from around Naomi's neck and pulls her up and onto my chest. We're in awe. Look at our baby! She's a girl, and she's beautiful.

It's time to deliver the placenta, which basically falls out. We get out of the tub, settle in the bed, and visit more with our new daughter. After a bit, I'm checked for tears—none, and not even any swelling! Naomi's turn next: she measures 21.5 inches long, 14-inch head circumference, and 7 pounds, 10 ounces. What a great baby! I tell my midwife that I might need to pee. She is amazed: many women don't feel like peeing for quite a while. But I did, and it was no problem.

By about one thirty in the afternoon we're all winding down, and I want our team to get going to miss the worst of the traffic back into the city. They cleaned up and left us with our new daughter. We tried to rest, but honestly, we mostly just stared at her.

This birth went incredibly well and was a healing experience for both my husband and myself, giving us renewed respect and confidence in my body's ability to sustain and bring new life into the world. We are so grateful to have been allowed the opportunity to experience, through our careful choice of the right midwife and location, a completely natural birth with no medical interventions. It was just what we needed.

Simone's Story

I'M A STUDENT MIDWIFE and my labor was the sixty-eighth I had attended. After about seven hours of active laboring in a birth pool, I delivered my baby on hands and knees on the couch. My birth was very quiet, calm, and deliciously pain-free. I heard my little one cry. After the few moments I needed to collect myself, I reached one arm down through my legs and patted around, asking "Where's my son?"

The midwife helped pass him through my legs and into my arms. I looked down at my baby and thought, "Huh, so this one's mine." The immediate postpartum was uneventful. My baby latched himself on within ten minutes of birth and there he stayed until the newborn exam. The student midwife took my son to a heating pad on the floor. Everyone was crowded around him, his father, both grandmothers, and the midwives. I got up to take a shower, calling behind me, "If there is anything abnormal, let me know." There wasn't.

On the third day, I woke up, looked at my baby, and I started crying uncontrollably. I felt so terribly guilty that for a good part of the past nine months, I had resented my son for the permanent tie he created between his father and me. His father was emotionally abusive and our relationship had been deteriorating slowly until it ended in flames the day before I went into labor.

I continued to feel guilty because in most every birth story that a mother will tell to a pregnant woman, no matter how horrific or tragic the labor, the ending is always the same: "And then I saw my baby and I fell instantly in love. I had never loved anyone so much in my life." Sure, I cared for my baby. I nursed him. I cuddled him. I changed his diaper. But it just felt like he was this baby that I was looking after.

At my three-week visit with my midwife, she asked if I had fallen in love with my baby. Upon seeing the look on my face, she added that some women fall instantly in love with their babies while for others it takes a couple of weeks. That made me instantly feel better and less guilty. She was right, too. I fell totally in love with my baby just over a month after he was born and never looked back.

Brenda's Story

I GUESS THIS STORY starts even before I was due. We all worried that this baby would not wait until my dear friend and doula arrived from Illinois to be with us. Her presence was so very important to me. But January 28 arrived and so did Jan, my doula-friend. No labor.

My due date arrives two days later, and nothing happens. At my next appointment, I ask to have my membranes stripped (where the midwife separated the sac from the cervix), but it doesn't do anything. The next week, we head out to meet our midwife and have a non-stress test. I'm fine, Baby sounds good, and I'm even having some contractions. I asked to have my membranes stripped again and that increases my cramps. As I shopped at Safeway later that day, I worried that my water would break in the dairy aisle.

No such luck. Time is ticking away and my doula-friend Jan has to fly home on Sunday! We decide to try castor oil to self-induce on Friday. I take two doses, both of which stay down for an hour and a half and then come back up. But no labor. I've also been taking homeopathic *Caulophyllum*, and who knows if that has done anything?

Around two thirty in the morning on Sunday, I'm having some bloody show and the cramps are getting stronger. My last two labors were quick, so I get excited, thinking things are picking up. I wake up Jan and then page the midwives. They decide to head over to the house, playing it safe rather than sorry.

By eight, I decide to put my music on and hang out in my room. Labor seems to be finally getting active, but when my daughters get up, I have a hard time letting go and letting the birth energy flow. Putting down the Mommy Mantle is very hard. There I am, contracting every five minutes, needing to lean over and moan slightly through them, but also making chocolate milk, getting bowls of cereal, turning on a cartoon, and trying to find treasured toys.

My mom, who is now officially a saint, leaves with the girls. I get in the tub, which feels nice. Looking at the water, I begin to grill Jan about her tub-cleaning skills, because I was sure I saw wads of cat hair floating in the water. Laborland is a strange place, where you see all sorts of strange things. I haven't been in the tub that long but I just can't stand it any longer, so I get out and labor on the toilet. Contractions are so intense at this point that each one is a struggle to get through without falling into tears. But now it's almost eleven and I'm thinking, "Why the hell haven't I had this baby by now? What the hell kind of position is she in? This is just taking so long!"

Jan called our friend Jennifer to step in as doula since her plane leaves today. At this point, I hear her telling me all this but I cannot cope with the meaning or even try to understand. I let it flow over me as she talks. When Jennifer arrives, I almost can't greet her, because to greet her is to let the reality of my greatest friend leaving become true.

I'm still on the toilet and Jennifer seamlessly moves in to take over holding my hands and talking me through contractions. I find the immense power of the contractions overwhelming and struggle to breathe and flow with them but Jennifer quietly tells me to soften my face, soften my bottom, and breathe down into them. It helps and I softly "OH" through several more while sitting on my toilet.

Back in my room I use the side of the crib as a kind of support, standing between contractions and squatting down and rocking during them. Jennifer is beside me reminding me to flow with them, to be loose and open. It is so difficult; each contraction is sharp with pain on my pubic bone and now my sacrum is starting to scream with the pressure of her head on it. I struggle to stay with the pains and find that zone where I can rock and moan trancelike through them. Jennifer's words are helping me remember to let go and trust not just in my body but in the force and energy of birth. I'm not really happy about doing it, but I try.

Each contraction is now taking me to tears. When I finish the next contraction, I say, "I don't think this is working." I hear someone asking, "What do you think is not working about it?" Someone suggests getting checked so we can find out where we are in the process. I just want to lie down and rest. I want my legs to stop shaking and to have a moment. I realize I don't like this slower labor. There's too much time to think between contractions. I like being in labor hard and fast, with no time for words or thoughts.

I move to the bed and suddenly my daughter Maren appears in front of me and strokes my face and gives me a sweet kiss. I am too deep in labor, and though I see her, it is like looking through a fish tank full of murky water. She says something to me and I whisper something back. I don't even know if I am making real words now.

Then Jan is there and she leans down to say she has to leave. She breaks and I can hear her sob. I want to hug her and say something to make this better. I want to suddenly pop the baby out but I am hanging on by a slim cord and I say, "Can't cry right now." I know she understands what I mean by that. Then she is gone.

For a minute, it is a dark place and I'm alone. How can I give birth without my doula-friend? Then the swell of a contraction comes and I am consumed again by the energy and force of this birth process. But this time, panic is rising as fast as the force of the contraction. I begin to gasp and cry in high-pitched tones verging on hyperventilation. Jennifer moves in on me then, putting her hands on my head and back, telling me in clear and quiet tones to breathe deeper, slower, and soften into the force. Okay, I think, and my tones immediately drop to the throbbing low pitch I've used before in birthing. Between contractions I look around and note that Jennifer is holding me, Don [my husband] is here, my midwife is here, the two students are here, and they continue to apply pressure to my back through each contraction. As with my other two births, I'm supported, cocooned, loved and listened to, and respected.

"Okay, so I can do this. I've done it before, even though this time sucks significantly harder. Just shut up and get it done," I tell myself. Seconds after I commit myself to getting out of the way of my process, a contraction swells up and at the peak, my water breaks with the force of a high-powered water gun. Now contractions are one atop the other and the real pushing begins. I'm making noises that sound like a bear or some other wild animal.

I'd like to stop making these ridiculously feral noises. However, it is as if they are not being made by me so much as my doppelgänger wild-woman and she doesn't give a shit. She is full of the force of birth. At that moment I feel my baby's head, all hard bone and round, as she enters the ever-forgiving birth canal. Someone puts a warm pack on my bottom and I'm comforted by it. Jennifer is rubbing my shoulders and it gives me peace.

I hear Don saying something and vaguely I register that Maren is in the room. The *me* part of me wonders if my feral wild-woman is scaring her, but the wild-woman doesn't give a shit about that either.

This moment feels like minutes, but who knows, it could be only seconds in which these things register. With the next contraction I am submerged or maybe it is elevated. "Elevated" sounds more right because now I am me no longer.

I am sound and light and absolute energy. It is as if a million suns are shining out from me and though my eyes are shut tight, I can literally see nothing but a blinding yellow. I can do nothing but make my feral sounds as my wild-woman pushes with the strength of all women. I am nothing but pure energy, and this force that worked on me, in me, has become me, and I feel my baby's head crowning. The burn of skin stretching has me reaching down with my right hand to put pressure on her head. "Please don't let me tear," I think. "Soften, let go," I think.

My midwife is giving me the play-by-play: "She is out to her eyes . . . [I'm still pushing] . . . she's out to her cheeks [still pushing] . . . now her chin . . . [still pushing] . . . her head is out." I am sure I'll have a moment to catch my breath now, but it doesn't come. I'm still pushing like a wild thing though I feel that nothing is happening. Each contraction has three or four waves of pushing, but through two contractions, I feel nothing happen.

"Great, she is stuck and we can't do the Gaskin maneuver because I'm already on my hands and knees," I think. I hear, vaguely as though they are talking to me from the living room, the midwives telling me to push, to really give it a good, hard push. I am pushing hard, but then comes my wild-woman again and she whips out those guttural sounds and out pop both of my girl's shoulders. "I hope her clavicles are okay," I think. Another solid push and she is out.

My bottom has had it; I have had it. I rest my head on a pillow. I look through my legs and see my baby, and then I'm turning over and grabbing for her. She is finally here.

I'm trying to push the placenta out but it's not ready yet. After quite a while and the passage of a large clot, the midwives have Don take AddyLou and put her skin-to-skin so we can get serious about this placenta. I can't seem to get any power to push it out while semi-reclining, so Jennifer helps hold me up in a squat. Finally after what seems like a really long time, the placenta comes out, whole and in some wacky way that the midwives refer to as "Dirty Duncan." This makes me think of Dunkin' Donuts, which makes me think "Mmmm, *doughnuts*," but I don't have any doughnuts to eat, dammit. Oh, and my bottom is intact but for a few little "skid marks," so hooray!

I've come to realize this birth was, for me, a transformation of self that I had not expected. Having been sure in my body's ability to give birth, I chose midwifery care and out-of-hospital birth years before, when I was pregnant with my first child. I had simple, uncomplicated experiences with both my first and second babies, and so my self-confidence and trust in the process of birth was undisturbed.

This third birthing challenged me. Physically, it was more intense and accompanied by nerve pain and muscle weakness. The labor was significantly longer than I had previously experienced, and my doula and dear friend who had accompanied us in the birthing of our two older children had to leave. It was a perfect storm of pressures, both internal and external, and more of me was required if I was to find safe passage.

Right after my water had broken, the heavy pressure of pushing was overwhelming me almost without a break. The electric pulse of nerve pain was shooting up my spine and down my right leg with every push and it felt like damage, like permanent harm was happening in my body. I had no power to change it. No one had the power to change it. I raised my head and through my closed eyes I could see the sun through my curtains, like a church's stained-glass, and I knew God had arrived in the room. I could feel the strength of love in the hands that helped me, I could feel the fire of it warming my skin. But mostly, I could feel how the trinity of my mind/body/spirit had opened up wanting a way to survive. I had been crying because some part of me was in despair of finding a way. And strangely, that was exactly when strength was illuminated.

It wasn't a gift being imparted but a reminder of where strength dwells: within me. I could do this, and I didn't have to do it alone. I had help. That day my midwives with their hands and hearts helped move me through each moment. My doulas, with their hands and words, were a constant warm rush of loving strength. My man, with his words and actions guarding the space took care of all within. My mother and daughters, with empathetic touches and words, helped as well. And finally, my baby, whose timeless movements and unflagging heart brought me such brightness. All of these special people were born through me that day, helping open me to a rebirth of myself.

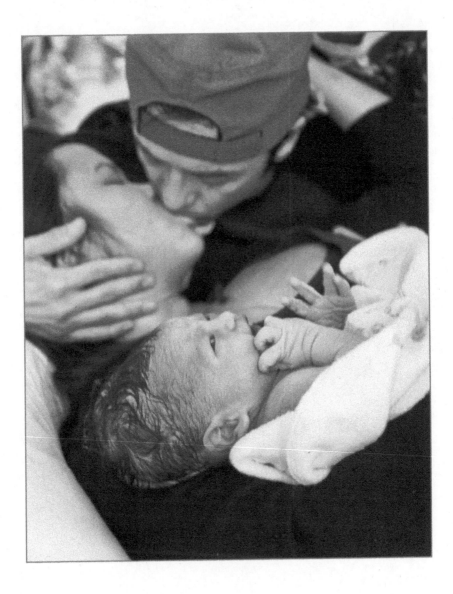

Questions to Ask During an Interview

BELOW YOU WILL FIND a general list of questions. It is not comprehensive; you will have questions that are specific to your history and your desires for your birth. You can use this as a guide or write your own interview questions. Consider taking notes on the midwife's answers so that you can look back at them later.

If the reason for asking the question is not readily apparent, we have added notes below the question *in italics* for you to refer to.

Questions About Her Business and Training

1. Are you licensed by the state? If not, why?

2. What are your fees?

    a. Do I pay a co-pay for each visit?

    b. What is included in the fees?

    c. What other costs might accrue?

    d. Are you open to a payment plan and, if so, what would that look like?

    e. What additional services or products do you offer that I might want to purchase?
    Among other options, this might include a birth tub, homebirth supply kit, or photographs.

    f. Do you bill to my insurance company?

3. How long is a typical prenatal visit appointment?

4. Do you typically run on time or late?

5. If I have a question, how long should I expect after I leave you a message for your return call?

6. What happens if you are at a birth or go out of town, and I have an appointment or go into labor?
   All midwives work with backup; ask who her backup is and if you will meet the backup midwife at any point during your pregnancy. It is not the norm to meet the backup unless it is very likely that this midwife will be out of town.

7. Tell me about how you got into midwifery.

8. Tell me about your education and training.

9. Do you participate in regular peer reviews?
   Peer reviews offer midwives the chance to reflect and learn from other midwives regarding every aspect of the care they provide. They are extremely beneficial learning experiences. If the midwife is participating in them, she is likely tied into her local midwifery community, which is very positive professional behavior.

10. Are you affiliated with a professional midwifery association and, if so, which one?
    If the midwife is a member of an association, you can look online to read about the kind of expectations they have for their members' practices.

11. Tell me about your services.

12. How would you describe your philosophy about midwifery and birthing?
    When all is said and done, you will have interviewed several qualified midwives. Which one spoke your language? Inspired you with her trust in mothers and babies? Made you feel safe? Listening to a midwife's philosophy provides valuable insight into these questions.

Questions About Prenatal Care

1. What are your expectations of clients during pregnancy?
   Does the midwife give you homework? Have diet restrictions? Expect you to keep a food diary or journal? Midwives often have these kinds of requirements because they have seen better outcomes with them.

2. How do you make decisions about tests and procedures, and which ones do you offer?
   The midwife should talk about shared decision making, informed consent, how she would feel if you declined a standard procedure, and if that would affect her care for you.

3. What resources do you have or recommend for us to prepare for home-birth?
   Many midwives have lending libraries of books and videos, and business cards for local services that they like to recommend.

4. What is your opinion about taking a childbirth education class?

5. What do your prenatal visits consist of?

6. Who will be at my prenatal visits, and what is their role?

7. Can I choose whether or not you use a Doppler during prenatal visits?
   Doppler is a type of ultrasound and it has not been proven safe in any evidence-based research. Many parents prefer the use of a fetascope or stethoscope.

8. If members of my extended family want to come to a prenatal visit, are you okay with that?

9. What are the things that would cause me to risk out of your care and a homebirth?

10. Who would you send me to if I risk out, and would you be with us for the birth as our doula?

11. Do you visit our home before I go into labor?

12. Will you offer us guidance in writing our birth plan?

Questions About Preparing the Home

1. What kind of supplies and equipment should I provide? Where should I purchase them from?

2. What kind of food should we have ready for your team?

3. We have a (dog, cat, bird, hamster, mother-in-law) living with us; will that be a problem for you?

If a midwife has allergies, it is her responsibility to bring allergy medica-tion, not yours to get rid of your pet.

4. What kind of map to our home should I give you?
Some programs give inaccurate directions on a consistent basis or are hard to read in the dark as we zip down the road. Most midwives will have a preference for how they want the map and directions made.

Questions About the Birth

1. When should I call you to tell you I am in labor?

2. At what point in my labor will you come to my home?

3. At what point after the birth do you leave?
The answer to this should be when both mother and baby are stable and have eaten. Some midwives stay longer, but none should plan on leaving earlier.

4. Tell me what kinds of things you do during labor. What should I expect?

5. Do you recommend that I hire a doula?

6. What kinds of supplies do you bring with you?

7. What is your view on waterbirth?

8. How do you handle delivery of the placenta?

9. How long do you wait before we cut the cord? What is your experience with lotus birth, and do you have an opinion about it?
At minimum the cord should be kept intact until it has stopped pulsing, indicating that your baby has received the full volume of blood from the placenta. "Lotus birth" is a term that describes leaving the cord attached to the placenta until it dries and breaks off. There are a variety of ways to pre-pare the placenta so that it does not have an odor during this period.

10. What happens if I tear? Can you suture me?

11. Have you handled emergencies with mothers and babies before?

12. What kinds of things might we transfer to the hospital for?

13. Will you come with me and stay with me if we transfer?

14. What is your transfer rate?

Questions About the Baby and Postpartum Care

1. Are you trained to resuscitate a newborn?
   Midwives should carry both current Neonatal Resuscitation and standard CPR cards.

2. What might happen during this time that we would need to transfer to the hospital for?

3. Do you do a newborn exam at home?

4. Are there any medications, tests, or procedures that you routinely do for newborns? Do we have the right to accept or refuse these?

5. How often do you visit us at home after the birth?

6. How often do we visit you at your office after the birth?

7. What happens at postpartum appointments?

8. When should we see a pediatrician?

9. How do we obtain a birth certificate?

Further Reading for the Homebirth Family

For parents or other grown-ups

Balaskas, Janet. *Active Birth: The New Approach to Giving Birth Naturally.* Boston: Harvard Common Press, 1992.

Block, Jennifer. *Pushed: The Painful Truth About Childbirth and Modern Maternity Care.* Cambridge, MA: Da Capo Press, 2008.

Buckley, Sarah. *Gentle Birth, Gentle Mothering: A Doctor's Guide to Natural Childbirth and Gentle Early Parenting Choices.* Berkeley, CA: Celestial Arts, 2008.

Davis, Elizabeth. *Heart & Hands: A Midwife's Guide to Pregnancy and Birth,* 5th ed. Berkeley, CA: Celestial Arts, 2012.

Davis-Floyd, Robbie. *Birth as an American Rite of Passage.* Berkeley: University of California Press, 2004.

Dick-Read, Grantly. *Childbirth Without Fear: The Principles and Practice of Natural Childbirth.* London: Pinter and Martin, 2005.

England, Pam. *Birthing from Within: An Extra-Ordinary guide to Childbirth Preparation.* Chicago: Partera Press, 1998.

Falk, Ursula Adler, and Gerhard Falk. *Grandparents: A New Look at the Supporting Generation.* Amherst, NY: Prometheus Books, 2002.

Gaskin, Ina May. *Ina May's Guide to Breastfeeding.* New York: Bantam, 2009.

———. *Ina May's Guide to Childbirth.* New York: Bantam, 2003.

———. *Spiritual Midwifery,* 4th ed. Summertown, TN: Book Publishing Company, 2002.

Goer, Henci. *The Thinking Woman's Guide to a Better Birth.* New York: Perigee Trade, 1999.

Klaus, Marshall H., MD, and Phyllis H. Klaus, CSW, MFCC. *Your Amazing Newborn.* Cambridge, MA: Lifelong Books, Da Capo Press, 1998.

Klaus, Phyllis, and Penny Simkin. *When Survivors Give Birth: Understanding and Healing the Effects of Early Sexual Abuse on Childbearing Women.* Seattle: Classic Day Publishing, 2004.

Romm, Aviva Jill, MD. *The Natural Pregnancy Book: Herbs, Nutrition, and Other Holistic Choices.* Berkeley, CA: Celestial Arts, 2003.

Siegel, Daniel J., MD, and Mary Hartzell, MEd. *Parenting from the Inside Out.* New York: Jeremy P. Tarcher/Penguin, 2004.

Simkin, Penny. *The Birth Partner—Revised 3rd Edition: A Complete Guide to Childbirth for Dads, Doulas, and All Other Labor Companions.* Cambridge, MA: Harvard Common Press, 2008.

St. John, Rose. *Fathers at Birth.* Portland, OR: Ringing Bell Press, 2009.

Vincent, Peggy. *Baby Catcher: Chronicles of a Modern Midwife.* New York: Scribner, 2002.

Wagner, Marsden, MD. *Born in the USA: How a Broken Maternity System Must Be Fixed to Put Women and Children First.* Berkeley: University of California Press, 2008.

Weed, Susan S. *Wise Woman Herbal for the Childbearing Year.* Ashcroft, British Columbia: Ash Tree, 1986.

Wiessinger, Diane, Diana West, and Teresa Pitman. *La Leche League International: The Womanly Art of Breastfeeding.* New York: Ballantine, 2010.

For children

Chasse, Malachi, and Jill Chasse. *Mommy's Lap: A Story of Sibling Love.* Charleston: CreateSpace, 2010.

Overend, Jenni, and Julie Vivas. *Welcome With Love.* San Diego: Kane Miller Books, 1999.

Resources for Childbirth Education and Support

Find out more about doulas here

Association of Labor Assistants and Child Birth Educators (ALACE)	www.alace.org
Birth Arts International (BAI)	www.birtharts.com
Childbirth and Postpartum Professional Association (CAPPA)	www.cappa.net
Doula Match	www.doulamatch.net
Doulas of North America (DONA)	www.dona.org

Find out more about childbirth education here

Birthing From Within	www.birthingfromwithin.com
The Bradley Method of Husband-Coached Natural Childbirth	www.bradleybirth.com
Hypnobabies	www.hypnobabies.com
HypnoBirthing	www.hypnobirthing.com
Lamaze International	www.lamaze.org
The Pink Kit	www.birthingbetter.com
Spinning Babies	www.spinningbabies.com

Resources for Higher Risk Mamas with Homebirth Hearts

Annette Rivlin-Gutman. *Mommy Has to Stay in Bed.* Charleston, SC: Book-Surge, 2006. Children's book explaining bedrest.

Kangaroo Mother Care, www.kangaroomothercare.com, support for parents of premature babies and information on skin-to-skin care for all babies.

March of Dimes, www.marchofdimes.com, a nonprofit foundation providing education and support around premature birth and birth defects.

Neo-Fight, www.neofight.org, phone and online peer-mentor support for parents with difficult pregnancies, premature or critically ill newborns, newborns with birth defects, or those who experience the death of a child shortly after birth.

Sidelines, www.sidelines.org, a nonprofit support group for parents experiencing high-risk pregnancies.

The Photos

THANK YOU TO THE many women who shared the photographs of their births. You are all beauties! Several were taken by professional photographers and we are grateful for their contributions:

Name: **KaetheJo Binder**

Bio: *KaetheJo Binder is a lifestyle photographer serving the greater Seattle area. She came to birth photography after the birth of her third child, and realized she had found her calling. While specializing in telling birth stories on film, she also enjoys shooting family portraits and other special events.*

Web site: www.kaethejo.com

Name: **Sindea Horste**

Bio: *Sindea Horste has been in business since 1995 as a birth and portrait photographer, and is also a birth and postpartum doula.*

Web site: www.sindea.org

Name: **Kyndal May**

Bio: *Kyndal May, CD(DONA), BDT(DONA), LCCE, is a storyteller and a facilitator, a confidence and community builder for expectant parents, doulas, and childbirth educators. To learn more about her birth doula workshops and childbirth education curriculum platform, visit her Web site.*

Web site: www.babybumpservices.com

Name: **Tiffany Perkins**

Bio: *Tiffany is a birth photographer located in the Seattle, Washington, area. She is also a mother to two beautiful boys and a wife to a wonderful husband. After receiving her BA from the University of Washington, Seattle, she decided to pursue photography and happened upon birth photography after photographing the birth of her nephew. While Tiffany enjoys all different forms of photography, photographing the birth of her nephew convinced her that birth photography would be her true passion going forward, and has since made it her main focus in photography.*

Web site: www.tiffanymae.com

Name: **Heather Puett**

Bio: *After beginning my journey as both a photographer and mother, birth photography seemed like a natural step. So many people spend thousands of dollars to capture wedding memories but spend essentially nothing on capturing the precious memories of their child's first moments. I want to change that and help capture those first moments of a newly formed family.*

Web site: www.heatherpuettphotography.com

Name: **Emily Stelea**

Bio: *A birth advocate since her teen years, Emily Stelea also began the study of art and photography at a young age. Following those passions she studied Women's Studies and Photography at the university level. Soon afterward she worked as both a birth doula and a portrait and commercial photographer. Combining these skills, her work now primarily focuses on birth photojournalism and newborn, infant, and child portraiture. Located in Southern California, Emily can be reached through her website: www .EmilyStelea.com.*

Web site: www.emilystelea.com

Acknowledgments

AGENT STEVE, YOU TAUGHT us not only how to write a book proposal but to greet each rejection with unwavering enthusiasm. You saw the diamond in the rough and encouraged us to shine. We have so enjoyed working with you!

Micki, somehow the universe threw us together for this journey. We couldn't ask for a better fit or a more wonderful and supportive editor. Your comments were always insightful and kind. We are so grateful that you were the midwife for our book!

Judie, you helped us organize our passionate ramblings into coherent paragraphs, and taught us the value of short sentences. Your heart is on every page.

We would never be where we are without all of the families who shared their stories and photos for this book. It would be incomplete without your words. You are the hope and potential of homebirth, and each of you are in our hearts.

A huge thank-you to all of the homebirth families we have had the pleasure to work with over the years as doulas and midwives. Thank you for sharing your lives and homes with us. It has been an honor.

Suzanne, our loving mentor and friend, you showed us the true meaning of faith in birth.

Carla, you taught us to never stop asking questions and to reframe every question into an opportunity for growth for every mother.

The ladies of Seattle ICAN, especially their fearless leaders past and present—Michelle, Verushka, Daisy, Marcia, and Sharon—you are the sisters of our heart. We have traveled a long journey together and you showed us who we could be as women, friends, doulas, and midwives. For the late nights, the long births, and the discovery of self: thank you.

For our Down and Dirty Birth Peeps: Health and wisdom have risen from the laughter, wit, and sharp insights you have all shared with us. Word.

For James Alexander Malcolm MacKenzie Fraser, and the friends who adored him with us, you infused us with happiness through the rough spots.

To the folks at Card Kingdom: Kim, you kept us fueled with hot tea and sandwiches, and to the Pinball Wizard who taught us how far a quarter can really go. And to Johnny Depp, who unwittingly sent us on our way.

From Jane: For my family

To my mother and father, you showed me what it means to be a parent, and waited patiently for me to write a book for at least thirty-five years. Dad, I wish you were here to see this. Pat, you support me every day in everything that I choose to do, regardless of how much it impacts our life. You never complain, never stop smiling, and never stop loving me. And finally to Anna, you birthed me into my mother-self, and you are my inspiration to change the world. I have loved every second of being your mom.

From Jodilyn: For my family

To my parents, you were the first to cheer my interest in writing and I am so thankful for your encouragement and support. Thank you to Ruben and Julie, who have loved me like a daughter for nineteen years. Benjy, we have loved each other through everything. Thank you for your support as I traveled around the world and back again, and for hiking through daily life with me. There's no one I'd rather be with on the trail. For my children: Julia, you made me a mother from the instant I gazed into your sweet eyes. You taught me everything good in the world. Sam, you were my miraculous VBAC and brought humor into the lives of all who knew you, I miss you so much. Jeffrey, your birth was full of light and joy. I loved meeting you—eager for the world in your first moments, your enthusiasm has never wavered. Loving the three of you has been the gift of a lifetime. Big hugs to my nieces and nephews, Aiden, Eli, Nora, Sema, Ruben, Mose, and Joelle, who remind me every day how fun it is to laugh with children.

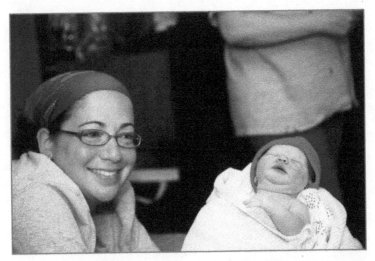

Jodilyn Owen with a baby received into her hands and heart.

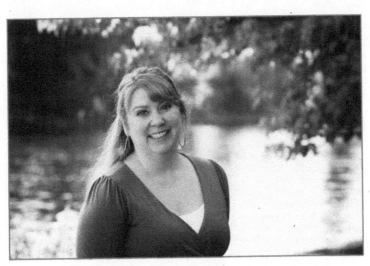

Jane E. Drichta: 650 babies and still smiling!

Notes

Chapter One: The Story of Homebirth

1. Karen Mullian, "Maternal Mortality: Fact or Fabrication," *Past Masters News* 3, no. 1 (Winter 2000).

2. Laurel Thatcher Ulrich, *A Midwife's Tale: The Life of Martha Ballard, Based on Her Diary, 1785–1812* (New York: Vintage, 1991), 170.

3. William Leishman, *A System of Midwifery: Including Diseases of Pregnancy and the Puerperal State* (Philadelphia: Henry C. Lea, 1873), 449.

4. Ibid.

5. Ibid., 448.

6. Jacqueline H. Wolf, *Deliver Me from Pain: Anesthesia and Birth in America* (Baltimore: Johns Hopkins University Press, 2009), 13.

7. *The Lancet* 376, no. 9738 (July 31, 2010): 303.

8. Eugene Declercq, et al., "Homebirth in the United States, 1989–1992: A Longitudinal Descriptive Report of National Birth Certificate Data," *Journal of Nurse-Midwifery* 40, no. 6 (1995): 480.

Chapter Three: Prenatal Care with a Homebirth Midwife

1. Arlie Russell Hochschild, *The Managed Heart: Commercialization of Human Feeling* (Berkeley: University of California Press, 2007).

2. D. W. Winnicott, *The Child, the Family, and the Outside World* (New York: Addison-Wesley, 1964/1987), 25.

Chapter Four: Midwifery Care, Homebirth, and the Mother's Community

1. Alice F. Freed, "Communities of Practice in Language and Gender Research," *Language in Society* 28, no. 2 (June 1999): 257.

Chapter Five: She Said, I Said, They Said—Communication

1. W. Rhys Roberts, "Rhetorica," *The Works of Aristotle*, volume XI, ed. W. D. Ross (London: Oxford University Press, 1924), 1358.

2. Wilbur Schramm, "How Communication Works," *The Process and Effects of Mass Communication*, ed. Wilbur Schramm (Urbana: University of Illinois Press, 1961), 5–6.

3. Centers for Disease Control and Prevention, "Prevention of Perinatal Group B Streptococcal Disease," *Morbidity and Mortality Weekly Report* 51, no. RR11 (2002): 1–22.

4. Amy Romano and Mayri S. Leslie, MSN, "Birth Can Safely Take Place at Home and in Birthing Centers," *The Journal of Perinatal Education*, 16 suppl. 1 (2007): 81S–88S.16.

5. P. A. Janssen, L. Saxell, L. A. Page, et al., "Outcomes of Planned Home Births with Registered Midwife Versus Planned Hospital Births with Midwife or Physician in British Columbia," *Canadian Medical Association Journal* 181, no. 6: 377–83.

6. Ibid.

7. Ibid.

8. A. de Jonge, B. van der Goes, A. Ravelli, et al., "Perinatal Mortality and Morbidity in a Nationwide Cohort of 529,688 Low-Risk Planned Home and Hospital Births," *BJOG: An International Journal of Obstetrics and Gynecology* 2009; doi:10.1111/j.1471-0528.2009.02175x.

9. Saraswathi Vedam, RM, FACNM, MSN, Sci D (h.c.); Laura Schummers, BSc, SM, and Colleen Fulton, BA, MA, *Bachelor of Midwifery.* "Homebirth: An Annotated Guide to the Literature." http://www.washingtonmidwives.org/assets/Home-Birth-Annotated-guide-to-the-literature-May2011.pdf; accessed 11/17/11.

Chapter Six: Your Expanded Pregnancy and Birth Team

1. Tiffany Field, "Pregnancy and Labor Massage," *Expert Review of Obstetrics & Gynecology* 5 (March 2010): 177–81.

2. Ibid.

Chapter Seven: Special Circumstances

1. Bruce Schneier, *Beyond Fear: Thinking Sensibly About Security in a Changing World* (New York: Springer, 2003), 26–27.

2. J. A. Martin, et al. "Births: Final Data for 2006," *National Vital Statistics Reports* 57, no. 7 (January 7, 2009).

3. Ibid.

4. V. C. Wright, et al., "Assisted Reproductive Technology Surveillance—2005," *Morbidity and Mortality Weekly Report*, 57, no. SS05 (June 20, 2008). "Assisted Reproductive Technology Surveillance," United States, 2003. Centers for Disease Control and Prevention, 02 May 2006. Web. 10 Nov 2011. www.edc.gov/mmmr/preview/mmwrhtml/ss5504a1.htm.

5. *Multiple Pregnancy and Birth: Twins, Triplets, & Higher Order Multiples: A Guide for Patients* (Birmingham, AL: American Society for Reproductive Medicine, 2004).

6. Traci B. Fox, "Multiple Pregnancies: Determining Chorionicity and Amnionicity," *Department of Radiologic Sciences Faculty Papers* (2006). Thomas Jefferson University, Philadelphia, PA.

7. J. A. Martin, et al., "Births: Final Data for 2006."

8. M. Habli, F. Y. Lim, and T. Crombleholme, "Twin-to-Twin Transfusion Syndrome: A Comprehensive Update," *Clinics in Perinatology* 36, no. 2 (June 2009): 391–416, x.

9. D. P. Cruikshank, "Breech Presentation," *Clinical Obstetrics and Gynecology* 29 (1986): 255–63.

10. J. Zhang, W. A. Bowes Jr., J. A. Fortney, "Efficacy of External Cephalic Version: A Review," *Obstetrics and Gynecology* 82 (1993): 306–12.

11. Andrew Kotaska, et. al., *The Society of Obstetricians and Gynaecologists of Canada Clinical Practice Guideline* no. 226 (June 2009): 557–58.

12. *Worldwide Sexual Assault Statistics* (Fairfax County, VA: George Mason University, 2005).

13. E. Sue Blume, *Secret Survivors: Uncovering Incest and Its Aftereffects in Women* (New York: Ballantine Books, 1989).

Chapter Eight: Homebirth After Cesarean

1. Carl Rogers, *On Becoming a Person* (Boston: Houghton Mifflin, 1961), 283–84.

2. B. E. Hamilton, J. A. Martin, and S. J. Ventura, "Births: Preliminary Data for 2010," *National Vital Statistics Reports Web Release* 60, no 2. (Hyattsville, MD: National Center for Health Statistics, 2011).

3. Ibid.

4. World Health Organization, "Appropriate Technology for Birth," *Lancet* 2 (1985): 436–37.

5. Geoffrey Chamberlain, Patricia Crowley, and Ann Wright, *Home Births—The Report of the 1994 Confidential Enquiry* by the National Birthday Trust Fund (Nashville: Parthenon Publishing, 1997).

6. Ibid.

7. Ibid.

8. S. Vause and M. Macintosh, "Use of Prostaglandins to Induce Labour in Women with a Caesarean Section Scar," *BMJ* 318 (1999): 1056–58. D. A. Miller, F. G. Diaz, and R. H. Paul, "Vaginal Birth After Cesarean: A 10-Year Experience," *Obstetrics & Gynecology* 84 (August 1994): 255–58.

9. "Vaginal Birth After Cesarean: New Insights," Structured Abstract. Rockville, MD: Agency for Healthcare Research and Quality, March 2010.

10. D. A. Miller, F. G. Diaz, and R. H. Paul, "Vaginal Birth After Cesarean: A 10-Year Experience."

11. K. M. Sweeten, et al., "Spontaneous Rupture of the Unscarred Uterus," *American Journal of Obstetrics & Gynecology* 172 (1995): 1851–55. D. A.

Miller et al., "Intrapartum Rupture of the Unscarred Uterus," *Obstetrics & Gynecology* 89 (1997): 671–73.

12. M. B. Landon, et al., "Risk of Uterine Rupture with a Trial of Labor in Women with Multiple and Single Prior Cesarean Delivery," *Obstetrics & Gynecology* 108 no. 1 (2006): 12–20.

13. "Vaginal Birth After Cesarean: New Insights," Structured Abstract.

14. Ibid.

15. Ibid.

16. Ibid.

Chapter Nine: The Big Ten

1. M. Malhotra, J. B. Sharma, S. Batra, et al., "Maternal and Perinatal Outcome in Varying Degrees of Anemia," *International Journal of Gynecology & Obstetrics* 79 (2002): 93–100.

2. E. J. Corwin, L. E. Murray-Kolb, and J. L. Beard, "Low Hemoglobin Level Is a Risk Factor for Postpartum Depression," *Journal of Nutrition* 133 (2003): 4139–42.

3. Bruce W. Hollis and Carol L. Wagner, "Nutritional Vitamin D Status During Pregnancy: Reasons for Concern," *Canadian Medical Association Journal* 174, no. 9 (April 25, 2006): 1287–90.

4. Magdalena Grundmann and Frauke von Versen-Hoeynck, "Vitamin D—Roles in Women's Reproductive Health?" *Reproductive Biology and Endocrinology* 9 (2011): 146, doi:10.1186/1477-7827-9-146.

5. S. H. Stein and D. A. Tipton, "Vitamin D and Its Impact on Oral Health—an update," *Journal of the Tennessee Dental Association* 91, no. 2 (Spring 2011): 30–33, quiz 34–35.

6. Michael F. Holick, MD, PhD, "Vitamin D Deficiency," *New England Journal of Medicine* 357 (2007): 266–81.

7. T. Bui and S. Christin-Maître, "Vitamin D and Pregnancy," *Ann Endocrinol* (Paris) 72 suppl. 1 (October 2011): S23–28.

8. C. S. Kovacs, "Vitamin D in Pregnancy and Lactation: Maternal, Fetal, and Neonatal Outcomes from Human and Animal Studies," *American Journal of Clinical Nutrition* 88, no. 2 (August 2008): 520S–528S.

9. C. R. Gale, S. M. Robinson, N. C. Harvey, et al., "Maternal Vitamin D Status During Pregnancy and Child Outcomes," *European Journal of Clinical Nutrition* 62 (2008): 68–77.

10. B. W. Hollis, D. Johnson, T. C. Hulsey, et al., "Vitamin D Supplementation During Pregnancy: Double-Blind, Randomized Clinical Trial of Safety and Effectiveness," *Journal of Bone and Mineral Research* 26, no. 10 (October 2011): 2341–57, doi:10.1002/jbmr.463.

11. Institute of Medicine, Food and Nutrition Board, *Dietary Reference Intakes for Calcium and Vitamin D* (Washington, DC: National Academy Press, 2010).

12. Ibid. D. Wolpowitz and B. A. Gilchrest, "The Vitamin D Questions: How Much Do You Need and How Should You Get It?" *Journal of the American Academy of Dermatology* 54 (2006): 301–17.

13. G. F. Chávez, J. Mulinare, and L. D. Edmonds, "Epidemiology of Rh Hemolytic Disease of the Newborn in the United States," *Journal of the American Medical Association* 265, no. 24 (June 26, 1991): 3270–74.

14. Ibid.

15. RhoGAM product label, including clinical trial data.

16. B. J. Stoll, "Blood Disorders" in R. M. Kliegman, R. E. Behrman, H. B. Jenson, and B. F. Stanton, eds., *Nelson Textbook of Pediatrics*, 18th ed. (Philadelphia, PA: Saunders Elsevier, 2007): chapter 103.

17. J. R. Verani, L. McGee, and S. J. Schrag, "Prevention of Perinatal Group B Streptococcal Disease—Revised Guidelines from CDC, 2010," *Morbidity and Mortality Weekly Report* 59 (November 19, 2010): 1–36. ACOG, "ACOG Committee Opinion No. 485: Prevention of Early-Onset Group B Streptococcal Disease in Newborns," *Obstetrics & Gynecology* 117, no. 4 (April 2011): 1019–27.

18. C. V. Towers, G. Padilla, et al., "Potential Consequences of Widespread Antepartal Use of Ampicillin," *American Journal of Obstetrics & Gynecology* 179, no. 4 (1998): 879–83.

19. T. B. Hyde, T. M. Hilger, et al., "Trends in Incidence and Antimicrobial Resistance of Early-Onset Sepsis: Population-Based Surveillance in San Francisco and Atlanta," *Pediatrics* 110, no. 4 (2002): 690–95.

20. H. C. Chen, M. D. Chang, and T. J. Chang, (1985) "Antibacterial Properties of Some Spice Plants Before and After Heat Treatment" (English translation of Chinese article), *Zhonghua Min Guo Wei Sheng Wu Ji Mian Yi Xue Za Zhi* 18: 190–95.

21. Centers for Disease Control and Prevention, "Prevention of Perinatal Group B Streptococcal Disease," *Morbidity and Mortality Weekly Report* 51 no. RR11 (2002): 1–22.

22. F. Facchinetti, F. Piccinini, S. Mordini, and A. Volpe, Department of Gynecology, Obstetrics and Pediatric Sciences, University of Modena and Reggio Emilia, Italy, "Chlorhexidine Vaginal Flushings Versus Systemic Ampicillin in the Prevention of Vertical Transmission of Neonatal Group B Streptococcus, at Term," *Journal of Maternal-Fetal and Neonatal Medicine* 11 no. 2 (February 2002): 84–88.

23. "Prevention of Perinatal Group B Streptococcal Disease."

24. Anne Frye, *Understanding Diagnostic Tests in the Childbearing Year: A Holistic Approach,* 7th ed. (Portland, OR: Labrys, 2007), 420.

25. Ibid.

26. K. E. Remsberg, R. E. McKeown, K. F. McFarland, and L. S. Irwin, "Diabetes in Pregnancy and Cesarean Delivery," *Diabetes Care* 22, no. 9 (September 1999): 1561–67.

27. Xilin Yang, Bridget Hsu-Hage, Hong Zhang, et al., "Women With Impaired Glucose Tolerance During Pregnancy Have Significantly Poor Pregnancy Outcomes," *Diabetes Care* 25 (September 2002): 1619–24.

28. G. G. Nahum and H. Stanislaw, "Ultrasonographic Prediction of Term Birth Weight: How Accurate Is It?" *American Journal of Obstetrics & Gynecology* 188 (2003): 566–74.

29. D. J. Rouse, J. Owen, R. L. Goldenberg, and S. P. Cliver, "The Effectiveness and Costs of Elective Cesarean Delivery for Fetal Macrosomia Diagnosed by Ultrasound," *Journal of the American Medical Association* 276 (1996): 1480–86.

30. Anne Frye, *Understanding Diagnostic Tests in the Childbearing Year: A Holistic Approach,* 7th ed. (Portland, OR: Labrys, 2007), 440.

31. Jeannet Lauenborg, Torben Hansen, Dorte Møller Jensen, et al., "Increasing Incidence of Diabetes After Gestational Diabetes: A Long-Term Follow-up in a Danish Population," *Diabetes Care* 27 (May 2004): 1194–99.

32. Samantha F. Ehrlich, Monique M. Hedderson, Juanran Feng, et al., "Change in Body Mass Index Between Pregnancies and the Risk of Gestational Diabetes in a Second Pregnancy," *Obstetrics & Gynecology* 117, no. 6 (2011): 1323–30.

33. A. M. Barbosa, A. Dias, G. Marini, et al., "Urinary Incontinence and Vaginal Squeeze Pressure Two Years Post-Cesarean Delivery in Primiparous Women with Previous Gestational Diabetes Mellitus," *Clinics* (Sao Paulo) 66, no. 8 (2011): 1341–46.

34. HAPO Study Cooperative Research Group, "The Hyperglycemia and Adverse Pregnancy Outcome (HAPO) Study," *International Journal of Gynecology & Obstetrics* 78 (2002): 69–77.

35. Anne Frye, *Understanding Diagnostic Tests in the Childbearing Year: A Holistic Approach.*

36. Kai J. Bühling, Tessa Winkel, Christiane Wolf, et al., "Optimal Timing for Postprandial Glucose Measurement in Pregnant Women with Diabetes and a Non-Diabetic Pregnant Population Evaluated by the Continuous Glucose Monitoring System (CGMS®)," *Journal of Perinatal Medicine* 33, no. 2 (March 2005): 125–31.

37. International Expert Committee, "International Expert Committee Report on the Role of the A1c Assay in the Diagnosis of Diabetes," *Diabetes Care* 32 (2009): 1327–34.

38. Stephen A. Walkinshaw, "Dietary Regulation for 'Gestational Diabetes'" *Cochrane Review* in The Cochrane Library, Issue 3 (Oxford: Update Software, 2000).

39. A. Khan, M. Safdar, et al., "Cinnamon Improves Glucose and Lipids of People with Type 2 Diabetes," *Diabetes Care* 26 (2003): 3215–18.

40. J. W. Anderson, MD, FACN, K. M. Randles, et al., "Carbohydrate and Fiber Recommendations for Individuals with Diabetes: A Quantitative

Assessment and Meta-Analysis of the Evidence," *Journal of the American College of Nutrition* 23, no. 1 (February 2004): 5–17.

41. B. Vaidya, S. Anthony, M. Bilous, et al., "Detection of Thyroid Dysfunction in Early Pregnancy: Universal Screening or Targeted High-Risk Case Finding?" *Journal of Clinical Endocrinology & Metabolism* 92 (2007): 203–207.

42. R. M. Calvo, E. Jauniaux, B. Gulbis, et al., "Fetal Tissues Are Exposed to Biologically Relevant Free Thyroxine Concentrations During Early Phases of Development," *Journal of Clinical Endocrinology & Metabolism* 87 (2002): 1768–77. B. Contempré, E. Jauniaux, R. Calvo, et al., "Detection of Thyroid Hormones in Human Embryonic Cavities During the First Trimester of Pregnancy," *Journal of Clinical Endocrinology & Metabolism* 77 (1993): 1719–22.

43. B. Stuckey, G. Kent, L. Ward, et al., "Postpartum Thyroid Dysfunction and the Long-Term Risk of Hypothyroidism: Results from a 12-Year Follow-up Study of Women with and without Postpartum Thyroid Dysfunction," *Journal of Clinical Endocrinology & Metabolism* (Oxford). (February 23, 2010): 1365–2265.

44. K. Duckitt and D. Harrington, "Risk Factors for Pre-eclampsia at Antenatal Booking," Canadian Task Force on Preventative Health Care, "Prevention of Pre-eclampsia." *BMJ* 330 (March 10, 2005): 576, doi:10.1136/bmj.330.7491.576. Available at www.ctfphc.org/Abstracts/ch13abs.htm.

45. National High Blood Pressure Education Program Working Group on High Blood Pressure in Pregnancy, "Report of the National High Blood Pressure Education Program Working Group on High Blood Pressure in Pregnancy," *American Journal of Obstetrics & Gynecology* 183 (2000): S1–S22.

46. Ibid. B. M. Sibai, "Diagnosis and Management of Gestational Hypertension and Preeclampsia," *Obstetrics & Gynecology* 102 (2003): 181–92.

47. F. Milne, C. Redman, et al., "The Preeclampsia Community Guideline (PRECOG)," *BMJ* 330 (March 2005): 576, doi:10.1136/bmj.330.7491.576.

48. L. Duley, D. J. Henderson-Smart, S. Meher, and J. F. King, "Antiplatelet Agents for Preventing Pre-eclampsia and Its Complications," *Cochrane Database of Systematic Reviews* (2007): 1.

49. C. A. Meads, J. S. Cnossen, S. Meher, A. Juarez-Garcia, et al., "Methods of Prediction and Prevention of Pre-eclampsia: Systematic Reviews of Accuracy and Effectiveness Literature with Economic Modelling," *NIHR Health Technology Assessment Programme* (Southampton, England), 12, no. 6 (March 12, 2008): 1–270.

50. National High Blood Pressure Education Program Working Group on High Blood Pressure in Pregnancy, "Report of the National High Blood Pressure Education Program Working Group on High Blood Pressure in Pregnancy," *American Journal of Obstetrics & Gynecology* 183 (2000): S1–S22. B. M. Sibai, "Diagnosis and Management of Gestational Hypertension and Preeclampsia," *Obstetrics & Gynecology* 102 (2003): 181–92.

51. D. Palevitch and L. E. Cracker, "Nutritional and Medical Importance of Red Pepper," *Journal of Herbs, Spices & Medicinal Plants* 3, no. 2 (1995): 67–70.

52. Rachel R. Pruyn Goldstein, Mary S. Croughan, and Patricia S. Robertson, "Neonatal Outcomes in Immediate Versus Delayed Conceptions After Spontaneous Abortion: A Retrospective Case Series," *American Journal of Obstetrics & Gynecology* 186 (2002): 1230–36.

53. Xiaobin Wang, Changzhong Chen, Lihua Wang, et al., "Conception, Early Pregnancy Loss, and Time to Clinical Pregnancy: A Population-Based Prospective Study," *Fertility and Sterility* 79 (2003).

Chapter Ten: Labor and Birth at Home

1. N. E. Vain, E. G. Szyld, et al., "Oropharyngeal and Nasopharyngeal Suctioning of Meconium-Stained Neonates Before Delivery of Their Shoulders: Multicentre, Randomized Controlled Trial," *Lancet,* 364, no. 9434 (2004): 597–602.

2. K. Christensson, C. Siles, L. Moreno, et al., "Temperature, Metabolic Adaptation and Crying in Healthy Full-Term Newborn Infants Cared for Skin-to-Skin or in Crib," *Acta Paediatrica Scandinavica* 8 (1992): 488–503. E. A. Begum, M. Bonno, N. Ohtani, et al., "Cerebral Oxygenation Responses During Kangaroo Care in Low Birth Weight Infants," *BMC Pediatrics* 8 (November 7, 2008): 51.

3. Dr. Marshall Klaus and Ms. Phyllis Klaus, in their foreward to the film *Initiation of Breastfeeding by Breast Crawl*, sponsored by Unicef, WHO, and WABA, http://breastcrawl.org/video.shtml.

4. H. Varendi, R. H. Porter, and J. Winberg, "Does the Newborn Baby Find the Nipple by Smell?" *Lancet*, 344 no. 8928 (1994): 989–90 and "Attractiveness of Amniotic Fluid Odour: Evidence of Prenatal Olfactory Learning?" *Acta Paediatrica Scandinavica* 85 (1996): 1223–27. H. Varendi and R. H. Porter, "Breast Odour as the Only Maternal Stimulus Elicits Crawling Towards the Odour Source," *Acta Paediatrica Scandinavica* 90 (2001): 372–75.

5. V. Terzidou, A. M. Blanks, S. H. Kim, et al., "Labor and Inflammation Increase the Expression of Oxytocin Receptor in Human Amnion," *Biology of Reproduction* 84, no. 3 (2011): 546–52.

6. R. Manganaro, C. Mamì, A. Palmara, et al., "Incidence of Meconium Aspiration Syndrome in Term Meconium-Stained Babies Managed at Birth with Selective Tracheal Intubation," *Journal of Perinatal Medicine* 29, no. 6 (2001): 465–68.

Chapter Eleven: The Postpartum Period

1. S. J. McDonald and P. Middleton, "Effect of Timing of Umbilical Cord Clamping of Term Infants on Maternal and Neonatal Outcomes," *Cochrane Database of Systematic Reviews* 2, no. CD004074 (2008), doi: 10.1002/14651858.CD004074.pub2.

2. C. M. Chapparo, et al., "Effect of Timing of Umbilical Cord Clamping on Iron Status in Mexican Infants: A Randomised Controlled Trial," *Lancet* 367, no. 9527 (June 17, 2006): 1997–2004.

3. A. Kuegelman, A. Kessel, et al., "Immunologic and Infectious Consequences of Immediate Versus Delayed Umbilical Cord Clamping in Premature Infants: A Prospective, Randomized, Controlled Study," *American Journal of Perinatology* 24, no. 5 (May 21, 2007): 307–15.

4. S. E. Rey and G. H. Martinez, "Manejo Racional del Nino Prematuro," *Proceedings of the Conference 1 Curso de Medicina Fetal y Neonatal, 1981* (Bogota, Colombia: Fundacion Vivar, 1983, Spanish). Manuscript available in English from UNICEF, 3 UN Plaza, New York, NY, 10017.

5. N. J. Bergman and L. A. Jurisoo, "The 'Kangaroo-Method' for Treating Low-Birth-Weight Babies in a Developing Country," *Tropical Doctor* 24, no. 2 (1994): 57–60.

6. G. C. Anderson, E. Moore, T. Dowswell, and N. Bergman, "Early Skin-to-Skin Contact for Mothers and Their Healthy Newborn Infants," *Cochrane Database Systematic Reviews* in The Cochrane Library (Oxford: Update Software, April 2003).

7. K. Christensson, T. Cabrera, E. Christensson, et al., "Separation Distress Call in the Human Neonate in the Absence of Maternal Body Contact," *Acta Paediatrica* 84, no. 5 (1995): 468–73. A. N. Schore, "The Effects of Early Relational Trauma on Right Brain Development, Affect Regulation, and Infant Mental Health," *Infant Mental Health Journal* 22, no. 1–2 (2001): 201–69.

8. C. Townsend, "The Hemorrhagic Disease of the Newborn," *Archives of Pediatrics & Adolescent Medicine* 1894 no. 11: 559–62 in J. Birkbeck, "Vitamin K prophylaxis in the newborn: a position statement of the Nutrition Committee of the Paediatric Society of New Zealand," *New Zealand Medical Journal* 101 (1988): 421–22.

9. R. Malia, F. Preston, and V. Mitchell, "Evidence Against Vitamin K Deficiency in Normal Neonates," *Journal of Thrombosis and Haemostasis* 44 (1980): 159.

10. A. McNinch and J. Tripp, "Haemorrhagic Disease of the Newborn in the British Isles: A Two-Year Prospective Study," *BMJ* 303, no. 6810 (1991): 1105–1109.

11. Lauren Feder, *Natural Baby and Childcare* (Hatherleigh Press, Long Island City, 2006), 336–39.

12. Helen, Varney, CNM, MSN, DHL. (Hon.) FACNM, *Varney's Midwifery* (Sudbury, MA: Jones & Bartlett Publishers, 2004), 978.

13. "Pelvic Inflammatory Disease" Sept. 28, 2011. CDC. www.cdc.gov/std/PID/STDFact-PID.htm.

14. M. O'Hara, "Ophthalmia Neonatorum," *Pediatric Clinics of North America* 40, no. 4 (1993): 715–25. M. Hammerschlag, "Neonatal Conjunctivitis," *Pediatric Annals* 22, no. 6 (1993): 346–51. D. Zanoni, S. Isenberg, and L. Apt, "A Comparison of Silver Nitrate with Erythromycin for Pro-

phylaxis Against Opthalmia Neonatorum," *Clinical Pediatrics* 31 (1992): 295–98.

15. Canadian Paediatric Society, "Recommendations for the Prevention of Neonatal Opthalmia," *Canadian Medical Association Journal* 129 (1983): 544–45. American Academy of Pediatrics and the American College of Obstetricians and Gynecologists, *Guidelines for Perinatal Care*, 4th ed. (Chicago, IL: American Academy of Pediatrics, 1997).

16. A. S. Imsiragic, D. Begic, and S. Martic-Biocina, "Acute Stress and Depression Three Days After Vaginal Delivery—Observational, Comparative Study," *Collegium Antropologicum* 33, no. 2 (June 2009): 521–27.

17. M. W. O'Hara, D. J. Neunaber, and E. M. Zekoski, "Prospective Study of Postpartum Depression: Prevalence, Course, and Predictive Factors," *Journal of Abnormal Psychology* 93, no. 2 (May 1984): 158–71.

18. A. M. Llewellyn, Z. N. Stowe, and C. B. Nemeroff, "Depression During Pregnancy and the Puerperium," *Journal of Clinical Psychiatry* 58, suppl. 15 (1997): 26–32. C. T. Beck "A Meta-Analysis of Predictors of Postpartum Depression," *Nursing Research Journal* 45 (1996): 297–303.

19. C. Cohen, J. B. Pimm, and J. R. Jude, *Coping with Heart Surgery and Bypassing Depression: A Family's Guide to the Medical, Emotional, and Practical Issues* (Madison, WI: Psychosocial Press/International Universities Press, 1998).

20. N. Shields, M. Reid, H. Cheyne, et. al., "Impact of Midwife-Managed Care in the Postnatal Period: An Exploration of Psychosocial Outcomes," *Journal of Reproductive and Infant Psychology* 15 (1997): 91–108.

21. Michelle Bland, "The Effect of Birth Experience on Post-Partum Depression," missouriwestern.edu. clearinghouse.missouriwestern.edu/manuscripts/118.php, 2009.

Index